ADVANCE PRAISE FOR *THE PERFECT BODY*

"Lots of fun, and wonderful characters. My kind of book!"
—**Janet Evanovich**

"*The Perfect Body* is lean, lithe, and full of curves. If you like your amateur sleuths funny and feisty, you'll love Annie March."
—**Jane Waterhouse**
Author of *Graven Images*

"Matetsky's debut has it all: vibrant characters, a style that sings, and a plot that never tricks or cheats."
—**Sterling Watson**
Author of *Deadly Sweet*

"The perfect read: deliciously scary, funny, and full of heart."
—**Sandra Thompson**
Author of *Close-Ups*

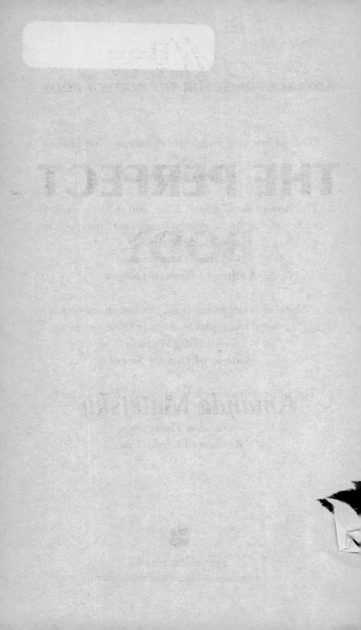

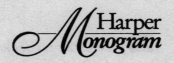

THE PERFECT
BODY

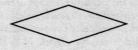

Amanda Matetsky

HarperPaperbacks
A Division of HarperCollinsPublishers

HarperPaperbacks
A Division of HarperCollins*Publishers*
10 East 53rd Street, New York, N.Y. 10022-5299

This is a work of fiction. The characters, incidents, and
dialogues are products of the author's imagination and are not to
be construed as real. Any resemblance to actual events or
persons, living or dead, is entirely coincidental.

ISBN 0-06-108490-5

HarperCollins®, 📚®, HarperPaperbacks™, and
HarperMonogram® are trademarks of HarperCollins*Publishers,* Inc.

Cover photo by Barnaby Hall/Photonica

First HarperPaperbacks printing: January 1997

Printed in the United States of America

Visit HarperPaperbacks on the World Wide Web at
http://www.harpercollins.com/paperbacks

❖ 10 9 8 7 6 5 4 3 2 1

For Harry, my nonfiction hero

Acknowledgments

I needed a lot of help during the writing of this book, and I got the best. I'm very grateful to the following people for their advice, interest, and encouragement: Deputy Inspector Patrick T. O'Connor, Commanding Officer of the Nassau County Police Academy, Nassau County Police Department; Ira Matetsky; Liza Clancy; Molly Murrah; Matthew Greitzer; Kathy Korth; D. Rose; Michele Anderson; Nikki Miller; Mary Reading; David Rawlings; Laura Bernikow; Sandy Thompson; Keith and Donna Kaonis; Tom and Santa De Haven. My husband, Harry Matetsky, was remarkably helpful and supportive, and my late father, Charles R. Murrah was nothing short of inspirational.

I especially want to thank my friends at Literacy Volunteers of America, Nassau County, Inc., who—without knowing it—gave me the determination and stamina to write the novel I had fantasized about for so long. In their company, and because of their brilliant example, I became a person who could set goals, make commitments, and see them to the finish line. And thanks to LVA-NC, I could not only write a book, but also teach somebody to read it.

Finally, I'd like to thank my agent, Pesha Rubinstein, who kept the faith when I had lost it, and my editor, Abigail Kamen Holland, who has a wonderful way with words.

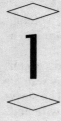

1

If I had known what was going to happen that night I would have locked myself up in the house right after supper with a good mystery novel and a pint of vanilla fudge ice cream. But I didn't have a clue. No raised hairs on the back of my neck, no tingling sensations on my skin, no nameless anxiety eating away at my sense of well-being. No visions or voices came to forewarn me that certain events, certain horrible events, would soon take place and change my life—change *me*—forever. So, instead of staying home as I should have, I put Linda Ronstadt's *Lush Life* album on the stereo, turned the volume up loud, and went about my usual Thursday evening activities like a woman without a worry in the world.

I took a quick shower and got dressed in my favorite black jeans and white cotton sweater. I sang "Falling In Love Again" with Linda while I put some color on my winter-pale face and tugged a brush through my thick, dark, shoulder-length hair. Taking a close look at myself in the bathroom mirror, I winked at my reflection. Not bad for a forty-three-year-old broad, I thought. Nothing wrong with Annie March that a ton of makeup and a bucket of hair dye can't fix.

For dinner I made some pasta marinara and a green salad, which I ate in front of my tiny tabletop TV watching the six o'clock news. Not a brilliant idea. The story about the Brooklyn man who murdered his wife and four children with a machete almost made me throw up.

Every night I watch the news while I'm eating, and every night I swear that I'm never going to do it again. But I know I won't be able to break the habit as long as I'm dining alone. I need the company of the people on the screen. I need to see them smiling and listen to them chatting about the events of the day. Even if they're chatting about rape and child abuse. I guess I'd rather be sick to my stomach than lonely.

After finishing dinner and cleaning up the kitchen, I headed for the bedroom to get all my stuff together. It wasn't a long walk. I live in a tiny ranch house that only a flea could get lost in—and some have, I imagine, since I have three cats. There's a small living room, an eat-in kitchen, one bathroom, and three little bedrooms, one of which I converted into an office. As a freelance magazine writer, I need a separate work area for my desk, computer, reference books, and clip files.

There's another room in my house as well, but I don't really think of it as a room. It used to be the garage until my late husband, Sam, turned it into his studio. It's kind of nice in there, actually—there's a skylight, an easel, a drawing table, and lots of art supplies—but ever since Sam's death five years ago, I only use the space for storage. I keep the door closed all the time and I don't go in there unless I have to. It hurts too damn much.

Grabbing my black tote bag full of books, paper, pencils, and note cards, I scooped the car keys off the dresser and hung my purse—a large sack of a thing that holds only my most important necessities and weighs as much as a watermelon—over my right shoulder. Then, snatching a light jacket off the coat rack by the front door, I left the house, as I did every Thursday evening around 6:30, and went to meet Philomena Tripp.

The drive from Rockville Centre, the Norman Rockwellesque Long Island town I live in, to the library in Hempstead where Philly and I always got together, only took about ten minutes. It might have been quicker if my car, a 1984 BMW with 150,000 miles on it, hadn't decided to do its impression of an old man with a limp and a bad cough. Luckily for me and my aging automobile, the south shore of Long Island doesn't have many hills.

As I crossed from Rockville Centre into Hempstead, the neatly trimmed lawns and lovely old homes gave way to drab storefronts and bleak apartment buildings, crumbling sidewalks and littered streets. I immediately became tense and watchful. It's like driving out of a quaint New England village straight into downtown Detroit. Well, that may be a slight exaggeration, but I checked to make sure that all the car doors were locked just the same.

When I got to the library I parked in the back lot as usual, to the left of the chain-link fence that separates the library lot from the lot of the Hempstead police station next door. One reason Philly and I didn't mind meeting there at night was the close proximity of the police station. It made us feel safe. Too safe, as it turned out. After I gathered my stuff together and got out of the car, I noticed that two of the lights in the area where I had parked were out, but I didn't bother to move to another spot.

I locked the car and began snaking around the other vehicles parked in my path through the lot. As I approached the walkway between the library and the police station, a few raindrops plunked on my head. Not wanting to get caught in a downpour later on, I dashed back to the car, unlocked the trunk, and took out my big red umbrella. Then I rushed back to the library without opening it.

Inside, my tension melted quickly in the warmth of the lights and the softness of the hushed and happy atmosphere. The small library was crowded—almost every seat was taken—and the air hummed with the murmurs of human voices and the whispers of turning pages. A group of high school kids sat giggling at a table near the front door, and off to the right, by the cook-book section, two men were having a friendly but rather loud argument about whether fried chicken should be coated in flour or corn meal. At least three of the patrons sitting in the long row of armchairs to the left were sleeping soundly. One of them, a middle-aged woman dressed in black sweats and wearing a Mets baseball cap, was snoring like a fat puppy.

I spotted Philly right away. She would have been hard to miss. With her dark brown skin, bleached-blonde punk hairstyle, bright red, rhinestone-studded glasses, and neon green raincoat, she looked more like an Andy Warhol painting than a real person. I grinned, as I always did when I first saw her. I walked over to the table where she sat hunched over her dictionary and I let out a low whistle. "If words were money," I said, "you'd be rich by now."

Philly looked up at me and her face split wide open with a smile. "How you doin', babe?"

"Just fine," I said, plopping down in the seat next to her. "How's it going with you?"

"Pretty good, 'cept I didn't get a chance to finish my homework on account of my car was stolen."

"What? Are you kidding?"

"No lie, girl. Somebody snitched it right out of the nursin' home parkin' lot while I was at work."

Philly had worked as a nurse's aide in the Hempstead Nursing Home for over fifteen years. She'd never progressed beyond this menial job because, up until four years before, when I became a Literacy Volunteer and started tutoring her, she didn't know how to read.

"Don't that beat all?" she said, stretching her big, lip-sticky mouth into a grimace. "Happened last Monday. Made me so mad I almost messed my pants. I was run-nin' all 'round the lot like a crazy girl lookin' for my ride, but it just wasn't there. Disappeared like Cinderella's buggy. Poof!"

"That's awful!" I felt like shouting, but I kept my voice down to a proper library whisper. "What did you do?"

"Oh, the usual stuff. Notified the police, filled out tons of forms, went to the Motor Vehicle Bureau and all. And I was able to fill in all the forms myself. That's thanks to you, girl. Nobody had to come with me, not one of my sisters, nobody. You would'a been proud of me." She combed several long fuchsia fingernails through her spiky blonde bangs and sat up straighter in her chair. "I was pretty damn proud of myself, if you want to know the truth."

"That's great, Philly. And I *am* really proud of you. You've come a long way."

"Yeah, but I've still got a long way to go, so let's get to work."

"Wait a minute!" I protested. "You haven't finished the story yet. Did they ever find your car?"

"No, and they never will. Must be busted up in a thousand pieces and all sold off by now. I bet there's people all over Queens drivin' around on *my* tires, revvin' up *my* engine, and listenin' to *my* radio."

"Did you have insurance?"

"Yeah, but it don't 'mount to much. After they get through evaluatin' this and depreciatin' that, you're left with nothin' but a bag of beans. Wouldn't be enough to buy a third-hand Pinto. It's a good thing Woodrow has his own car dealership," she said, referring to her husband of more than ten years. "He was able to get me a real good deal on a demonstration Sundance."

"Do you have the new car yet?"

"Sure thing. Got it the next day. Can't be without my wheels! I parked it behind the police station for safekeepin'." She slipped her neon green raincoat off her shoulders and tucked it over the back of her chair. Underneath, she was wearing a white uniform which gave off a faint scent of urine. When you empty bedpans all day some of the odor is bound to stick.

"Anyway," Philly continued, "I was so busy with all this junk that I didn't get to finish my homework. I put my new words into sentences and I wrote in my journal every day, but I didn't get 'round to the spellin' exercises."

"That's okay," I said, taking my notebook and a stack of flash cards out of my tote bag. "Let's start with the cards and go over the homework later."

"Oh, good!" Philly's black eyes began twinkling like the rhinestones on the frames of her glasses. "I love doin' the cards!"

She didn't have to tell me that. After four years of weekly two-hour lessons, I knew Philly's preferences well. I also knew exactly how she would behave while we were working on the flash cards. If she didn't know the word on the card, she would slump down in her chair and begin trying to read it in a very soft voice. Then, the closer she would get to decoding the word, the straighter she would sit and the louder she would speak. She never wanted me to tell her what the word was. She wanted to keep working on it and guessing at it until she got it herself. I took the card printed with the word "Fated" from the deck and held it out in front of her.

"Frisked," she whispered, slouched so low her chin almost touched the tabletop. "Fish . . . fished . . . friend . . . Fred . . ." She was stumbling and she knew it. Short words were the hardest for her, and she often had trouble with vowel sounds. But rather than slowing down and trying to sound out the word or just read a part of it as I had taught her, she speeded up. "French . . . fried . . . framed . . . freak . . . frap . . . farkle . . ."

She was really losing it. Her drooping shoulders slumped low over the table. But just as I was about to give her a little hint or some decoding direction, she seemed to get a grip on herself. "Frank," she muttered, raising her head a few inches. "Farmer," she said, uncurling her backbone and aligning it with the back of her chair. Then, straightening to full height and proudly stretching her chin up toward the ceiling, she gleefully shouted, "Farted!"

A sudden silence fell around us. The teenagers across the way stopped tittering and stared at Philly with wide-eyed wonder. A man at the end of the table snapped his head toward us in shock, and the old woman sitting to my right shot *me* an angry look. She quickly inched her chair away from mine and began sniffing the air with beaglelike concentration.

Philly and I looked at each other and, as she realized what she had just said—or, rather, *shouted*—her face twisted into a wad of amazement and embarrassment. Then we started laughing. And I thought we would never stop. Trying our best not to make too much noise, we chuckled and snorted and snickered and wheezed. We held onto our sides and doubled over in exquisite convulsions of pain. And all our efforts to contain ourselves only made our pleasure greater. Forbidden laughter, like forbidden sex, packs its own special intensity.

After what seemed to be an interminable period of time, we managed to put a lid on it and limp through the rest of our lesson. We went over all her homework, we worked on the -*ight* word pattern, and then I made flash cards of some of the words she stumbled over while reading an article in *Prevention* magazine. We were careful not to make eye contact because we both knew if we looked at each other we'd crack up again. I gave her the new word cards to study at home and put into sentences, plus a few other homework assignments. Then we packed up all our stuff and headed out to the parking lot together.

A hard rain had come and gone. Little rivers were running in the gutters; the streets and sidewalks glistened like oil slicks. Freshly washed, the damp night air smelled clean and sweet. Philly and I strolled along the pavement between the library and the police station, dodging puddles and laughing about the ill-*fated* flash card incident.

"See what a difference one little letter can make?" I told her.

She groaned, suddenly shifting gears from silliness to shame. "That one little letter made a total butthead out of me. I don't know why you waste your time with me, Annie. I'm so dumb it's dangerous!"

"Oh no, Philly!" I said quickly. "That's not true at all. If you take another look at what happened, you'll see that all you did was insert one wrong letter into the word. You got all *five* of the other letters *right*." One of the first things they teach new tutors at Literacy Volunteers is that, no matter how brave or cocky the students may act, most of them have very low self-esteem. Not being able to read can do that to a person. A good tutor will work to build self-confidence as well as reading skills. And I like to think of myself as a damn good tutor. Besides, there's nothing dumb about Philly. In some ways, she's smarter than I ever dreamed of being.

"Hey, girl!" Philly chirped, jumping over a big puddle in the middle of the parking lot. "You tryin' to tell me that I lost my seat on the Stupid Train?"

"I'm saying you never belonged on that train in the first place. Walk me to my car," I said, leading the way through rows of automobiles to the back of the lot, "and then I'll drive you over to yours. It's pretty dark back here. Creepy."

I knew Philly would think I was being a scaredy-cat—she'd called me that on more than one occasion. But I didn't care. I *was* scared. The May night felt misty and mysterious. Our footsteps made eerie echoes on the wet cement and something seemed to be moving in all the shadows.

When I got to my car I walked around to the rear. "I

just want to put my bag and umbrella in the trunk," I said, and Philly waited patiently by the front passenger door while I fished around in my purse for my keys. But as I leaned over to unlock the trunk I saw that it was already open. I must have forgotten to lock it when I came back for my umbrella. *Bad move, Annie.*

And when I opened the lid all the way I saw just how bad a move it had been. The trunk, which had been empty except for my umbrella, a flashlight, a pair of jumper cables, and an old beach towel, was now filled with a huge, heavy-duty, dark green plastic trash bag. And the bag itself was obviously filled with something big and bulky.

I grabbed my flashlight from the front left corner of the trunk, turned it on, and moved the beam of yellow light over the suspicious package. The opening of the bag was tightly sealed with a wide thickness of sturdy electrical tape. At first I thought somebody had done a major yard cleanup and, rather than lug all the weeds and branches out to the town dump, had decided to deposit the load in my conveniently open trunk. Then I wasn't so sure.

"Philly," I called out, "come here a second. Look at this! Somebody put something in my car!" Philly came around to the back and peered inside the trunk. I aimed the flashlight so she could see. "What do you think it is?" I asked her.

"Looks like a pile of old clothes," she said. Then she bent over and took a closer look. "Or maybe it's a dead body!" She made a wicked face in my direction and let out an exaggerated witch's cackle.

"Aagh! Don't even say such a thing," I backed away from the car.

"Only one way to find out." She bravely stretched out

her hand and poked the top lump of the package with her index finger.

I squealed. "Don't do that! What is it? What does it feel like?"

"Right here it feels like a plastic-covered cantaloupe. Lemme see what this part feels like," she said, gingerly poking at another lump in the bag. "This part feels like a eggplant. Hey! I know what this is," she said with certainty. "This here's a big sack of groceries!"

"Don't be silly. Why would anybody fill up a huge trash bag with groceries? And, even more to the point, why would they put it in my car?"

"Maybe they saw you go into the library and thought you looked hungry. You *are* kind of skinny, you know."

"Come on, Philly! Stop joking around. This is serious. I'm getting the creeps. I want to go home and I can't, not with that . . . that *thing* in my trunk."

"Well, there's only one thing left to do," she said. "We got to open this sucker up and see what's inside." With that she lifted up a fold of the green plastic and jabbed a hole in it with her long fuchsia thumbnail. Then she worked the fingers of both hands down into the hole and pulled in opposite directions until the plastic gave way and split wide apart.

"Good Lord have mercy," she said softly, standing back from the car and staring into the trunk.

"Oh no," I mumbled, moving closer to the car, holding the flashlight higher and praying to God that I wasn't going to see what I feared I was going to see. My prayers were not answered. There, in my trunk, curled up against the chill of the damp night air and the slick cling of the hideous green plastic, lay the naked body of a beautiful young woman.

She was lying on her right side, loosely curved in the

shape of a question mark. Her long, thick blond hair was coiled in damp snakes around her neck and shoulders. From where I was standing, one perfectly formed breast, with its perfect girlish nipple, was visible. She had a small waist, slender hips, rounded buttocks, and taut, smooth thighs. And she had no life in her at all. Her dark eyes were open and they stared blankly ahead at the vast nothingness her future had become.

I gasped and turned my head away. My brain kicked into the spin cycle and the parking lot turned into a whirlpool. To keep myself from passing out I took several deep breaths and focused my eyes on Philly's face. Tears were rolling down her cheeks. For a second I thought I was going to throw up, but then the nausea passed and I was left with just a hard cold stone of sadness in my stomach. And a gnawing tug of curiosity. "I wonder what killed her," I said, forcing myself to turn back to the trunk and look at the body again.

Even in the yellow glow of the flashlight, her skin looked gray. Both arms were bent in front of her and her hands were curled like claws. She was completely naked except for a gold charm bracelet and a pair of white, blood-spattered socks. I walked around to the left side of the trunk and trained the flashlight beam on the front of her body. That's when I saw the gunshot wound. The bullet had entered the very center of her chest, midway between her breasts and the tops of her shoulders.

To see where the bullet had exited the body, I had to walk around to the other side of the trunk and pull the green plastic further away from the girl's back. That's where the largest wound was. The bullet had blasted out through the spinal column, down near the waist and the tops of the hips. That's also where most of the blood was, brown and coagulated in the folds of the trash bag.

I couldn't believe how calm I was acting. My heart was pounding—pumping my own blood through my veins at an alarming rate—but there I was, walking around the trunk of my car examining a dead body with the cool detachment of a mortician. Philly was in shock—as much at my behavior, I think, as at the circumstances.

"Thank goodness the police station is right here," I told her. "Let's go over and get somebody." I unlocked the car door and shoved my tote bag, umbrella, and flashlight onto the back seat. I lowered the lid of the trunk, but didn't push it down hard enough for the latch to catch. I couldn't bear the thought of shutting that poor girl up in there again.

"I can't move," Philly said. "I'm stuck here like a tree."

"Do you want to stay with the body while I go get 'the fuzz'?" I don't usually talk like that. I just thought some dopey white jive might break the spell and make her smile.

"Are you crazy, girl? If I stay here there'll be *two* dead bodies by the time you get back." She turned in the direction of the police station and walked quickly away from the car. "'Sides," she said as I rushed to catch up with her, "you gonna need somebody to back up your story. They might think you havin' hallucinations or somethin'."

We dashed across the parking lot and mounted the cement steps to the station entrance. Inside the door and straight ahead was a kind of fenced-off area—a room separated from the tiny entrance foyer by an armpit-high counter with a swinging door. The place looked more like a post office than a police station. The lighting was very dim, and behind the counter were several desks, three or four chairs, lots of wooden cubby holes filled with bits of paper, and no people at all.

"Hello!" I called weakly. "Is anybody here?" Unless I'm angry, I find it hard to raise my voice. I looked around on the counter for something to ring or buzz, something like a hotel desk bell, but I couldn't find anything. "Hello!" I called again.

When nobody rushed out of the back rooms of the police station to answer my call, Philly let out with the most ear-piercing, crystal-shattering scream I'd ever heard in my life! I thought a siren went off in my head. It was a good thing I didn't have any wine glasses on me.

After her scream stopped bouncing off the walls, Philly cried out, "Help! Help! Murder! Murder!"

That did the trick. A door at the very back of the room opened halfway and a silver-haired man popped his head out. It was a huge head, the size of a basketball. The man gave us a quizzical look and then actually pushed the door all the way open and walked through it. He was tall and stocky and wearing a uniform—black pants, black belt, black tie, and a crisp, white short-sleeved shirt with a round emblem or badge on it. He sauntered over in our direction and faced us across the counter.

"Can I help you?" he asked with obvious disinterest.

I opened my mouth to speak, but before I could get a word out, Philly cried, "Mister! Officer! You got to help us! There's a dead lady outside in my friend's car!"

"Oh yeah?" he said, looking at Philly as if she'd just tumbled down from Jupiter. I don't know if it was because of her blonde hair, weird glasses, and wild raincoat, or just because she was black, but he seemed to doubt her words and regard her with little respect.

That really pissed me off. And, though I sometimes find it as difficult to speak my mind as I do to speak in a loud voice, I sprang to Philly's defense. "My friend has stated the case correctly," I said in the snottiest manner I could muster. "If you're not too *busy* with other matters, matters more important than the murder of a young woman, perhaps you will accompany us out to my car in the library parking lot. There you will find all the proof you need that Philomena has told you the truth, and," I added with a slice of sarcasm, "nothing but the truth."

He had a big head, but there wasn't much in it. "Is that so?" he said predictably. Then he looked around the room and scratched his massive jaw. "Wait here. I'll go get some backup."

Three hours later, I was still in Hempstead. It was after midnight and I was exhausted. The detectives who had been summoned to the scene from Nassau County Police Headquarters in Mineola had let Philly go home about an hour and a half earlier, after they realized there was nothing more she could tell them. She had offered to stay with me, but I convinced her to leave. She had to be at work at 6:30 the next morning, and I didn't have to be at work at all. Being the widow of a well-insured husband does have some advantages. Not many, but some.

I wasn't allowed to leave because *I* had discovered the body, the body was found in *my* car, and they had to go over every inch of my trunk looking for every possible clue or piece of evidence. I stood outside with the homicide detective in charge, Sergeant Eddie Lincoln, and answered his interminable list of questions. He wanted a minute-by-minute account of that evening, of course, but he also asked for a lot of details about my past—date and place of birth, marital status, maiden name, stuff like that. We stood and talked while the photographers, both still and video, lit up the entire taped-off area with special spotlights and recorded the gruesome scene on film.

The sergeant was kind of cute. Tall, sturdy, curly brown hair, and lots of freckles. He reminded me of K.O. Kelly, a main character in the Katy Keene comics I used to read as a kid. Standing outside with him sure beat sitting inside with Officer Obnoxious, the creep Philly and I first reported the crime to. Besides, I wanted to watch what was happening.

A team of guys from the Medical Examiner's office arrived in a white, unmarked ambulancelike van and made a thorough study of my car and the young woman's body. They dusted for fingerprints and collected bits of fiber and grit in tiny plastic pouches. Afterward, they lifted the poor girl out of the trash bag and out of my trunk. They zipped her up into another bag, strapped her onto a stretcher, then shoved her into the back of the van and whisked her away into the night.

"Where are they taking her?" I asked the sergeant, like a total nitwit. Where did I *think* they were taking her, to a picnic?

"To the morgue," he said with an almost straight face. Nice of him not to make fun of me or treat me like the idiot I was impersonating. "The ME—that's the medical examiner—will give her a good going-over, and then they'll keep her in cold storage until they find out who she is—I mean, was."

"How will they do that?" Another brilliant question.

"Somebody in her family will probably report her missing by the morning. She doesn't look like the type who'll stay a Jane Doe for long. Expensive gold bracelet, manicured fingers and toes."

"How do you know about her toes? She was wearing socks." Just call me Miss Marple.

"Her socks were removed and put with the other clothes they found stuffed in the bottom of the trash bag. The whole bloody mess, including the bag, goes to the MEO and then to forensics." He was being nice to me. He really was. He didn't have to answer all my dumb questions. I think he knew, in spite of my calm demeanor, that I was freaked out, fouled up, and terrified of driving home alone, in a car that had just been used as a coffin.

Little did I know that they had no intention of *letting* me drive home. "I'm afraid we're gonna have to impound your car," Sergeant Lincoln told me, "until we're sure we got all the evidence."

"Oh great! How am I supposed to get home?"

"Don't worry about that. They're almost finished here, and I don't have to stick around anymore. Come with me and I'll take you home in a squad car."

As we turned to walk across the lot, I took one last glance at my car. Relieved of its dreadful cargo, my still-open trunk looked oddly empty—very large and, strange to say, lifeless. There were no signs at all that the beautiful dead girl had ever been there. Not a single tuft of blonde hair, not the slightest trace of blood, not one pearly sliver of bone. Nevertheless, I knew that I would never again open my trunk—or *any* car trunk—without thinking of her.

The drive from Hempstead to Rockville Centre was quick and quiet. There were still a lot of questions I wanted to ask Sergeant Lincoln, but I just didn't feel like talking. Apparently he didn't, either. We rode most of the way in silence, listening to sporadic reports and intermittent static on the police radio. As we neared my neighborhood, I gave him directions to my house.

When he pulled into my driveway, I already had my house key in my hand. "Thanks for the ride," I said, opening the door of the squad car. "When do you think I'll be able to get my car back?"

"That's hard to say," he answered. "It all depends on how quickly the investigation goes, if the car has to be kept as evidence for a trial, or whatever. Could be a month. Might be longer. I would advise you to obtain some other means of transportation, for the time being at least."

"Okay," I said, too much in shock to protest. I gave him a befuddled smile, got out of the car, and closed the door.

Sergeant Lincoln quickly leaned over and rolled down the passenger window. "Oh, Annie? Uh, Mrs. March?" he called. I leaned down to see what he wanted. "I, uh, I forgot to inform you that we'll have to call you in to headquarters soon for further questioning." He paused, seeming embarrassed. "I've also got to tell you not to leave town."

"Why?" I asked, laughing. This was beginning to seem like a B movie. "Am I a suspect or something?"

"Well, no, not really. I mean, I don't think so. But I've got to ask you to stick around anyway. It's routine procedure. In eight cases out of ten, the person who discovers the victim's body turns out to be the murderer."

He gave me a little wave and began backing out of the driveway. I scuttled up to my front door and let myself in. As I hung up my jacket, I caught a glimpse of my face in the mirror above the coat rack. My mouth was gaping open like a forgetful old man's fly.

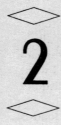

2

I was glad to be home, back inside my little house with my kitties, my books, my stereo, and my TV. I turned on the set in the bedroom for company. *Bringing Up Baby* with Cary Grant and Katharine Hepburn was on, but I couldn't relax and lose myself in the film until I searched through the whole house, checking every corner and closet for gun-toting intruders.

I found a few visitors but they were the peaceful, spiritual kind. The ghost of my dear husband followed me from room to room, patting my back, stroking my hair, and telling me not to worry. The voice of my long-departed mother called to me from the kitchen, telling me to calm down, that everything would be all right. I wanted to believe them and sink into the reassuring comforts of my home, but the specter of the beautiful dead girl I had found in my car was curled up like a fetus in the middle of my living room carpet, making me feel anything but cozy.

I gave the kitties a snack, washed my face, and quickly changed into my sleeping uniform—an ancient white-cotton T-shirt printed with the Rolling Stones's stuck-out-tongue logo. I checked to make sure all the doors were locked. I turned on the outside lights and turned off most of the inside lights. And then I went, with a clenched stomach and a deep sense of disquiet, to bed.

I couldn't have fallen asleep if a tanker-load of morphine had been pumped into my veins. Lying rigid as driftwood on my big beach of a bed, I braced myself and waited for the memories to crash over me. I knew they would come. And once they began pounding on the shore of my consciousness, they engulfed me as thoroughly and relentlessly as the waves of cold blue light from the television. I was powerless to stop the process. I could only lie there, thinking the unthinkable, bearing the unbearable. Five years had passed, but the images and emotions were as strong and fresh as ever. . .

It was a Tuesday night and Sam had called from the city to say he'd be home late, that he had to design a new cover for one of his company's magazines in time for a nine o'clock meeting the next morning. I didn't mind too much. I'd been working all day on a boring article about nutrition and exercise for *Self* magazine, so I was tired. To make up for the time I'd spent writing about fresh fruits and vegetables, I had a salami sandwich and a can of beans for dinner. Then I watched my favorite old movie, *All About Eve*, for about the eightieth time on the American Movie Classics channel.

By ten o'clock, when Sam still hadn't come home or called, I started to worry. Normally, he would have spoken to me two or three times by then. We used to joke that he would save himself a lot of time and trouble by having a phone permanently grafted onto his ear. For him *not* to have called was totally unnatural. I phoned his office several times, but there was no answer. By eleven, I was pacing around the living room like a lunatic, peering anxiously through the venetian blinds, praying with all my might for his headlights to appear in the driveway.

Finally, around one o'clock in the morning, a pair of headlights did appear in the driveway. Only they weren't Sam's. They belonged to the patrol car that brought the tall, thin uniformed policeman to my door to tell me, in a small, shaking voice, that my husband had been murdered. In his office. At his desk. Shot through the neck by an unknown assailant. Died instantly. Motive: robbery.

Sam's wallet had been taken and many of the drawers in the twenty-or-so other desks at the small publishing company had been ransacked. A woman working in the insurance office down the hall had also been shot. In the face. Not dead, but close to it. Purse gone. No leads. No suspects. No witnesses except the victim, if she survived.

I never summoned the tall, thin officer into the house. I stood frozen at the front door while he gave me the grim details. His words whipped through my brain like a hot, dry wind. He said NYPD detectives would contact me soon; I said okay. He asked me if I would be all right; I said yes. He told me I should call somebody to come stay with me; I said I would. He said he was sorry; I said thanks. Then he turned and headed down the front steps to the car. I closed the door, locked it, sank to my knees on the carpet, and passed out in a heap at the foot of the coffee table.

When I came to, Groucho—the cat Sam had picked from a box of free kittens outside the grocery store and brought home in his coat pocket—was snuggled up next to my belly, snuffling noisily into the folds of my blue flannel robe. There was a lump on my forehead the size of an egg—from crashing into the coffee table, I guess—and I didn't know what day or time it was. I made no attempt to find out, either. I just called my father up, told him what had happened, and asked him to come quickly.

My father dealt with the detectives and identified the body. I went to bed. And in bed I stayed. Except for going to the bathroom, making rare trips to the kitchen for something to eat or drink, and going to the funeral—which my father arranged with the help of Sam's sister—I stayed in bed for two weeks. I got out of bed when my father left and returned to his own apartment in Port Washington. But I still didn't leave the house. Not for three more weeks. I didn't leave the house until all I had left to eat was a can of creamed corn and three stale saltines. I was out of cat food, too.

They never found out who killed Sam or the lady from the insurance company, who never regained consciousness and died two days after the shooting. And to this day I still wonder who did it. Sometimes, when I'm walking down the street, especially if I'm in the city, and I see a man with a greedy face, or a man who's in a suspicious hurry, or a man with cruel-looking clothes, I wonder if it's *Him*. I wonder if I've just passed within spitting distance of the monster who ended my husband's life and demolished mine. Then I wonder if the killer has any remorse. And then I wonder if he even *remembers* killing my husband. The only thing I *don't* wonder about is what I would do if they ever caught the murderer and put me in a room with him with a loaded pistol in *my* hand.

Would I pull the trigger? In a heartbeat.

When the light from outside became brighter than the light from the television, I got out of bed. I put up a small pot of coffee and ate a banana while it perked. I guzzled down one quick cup and, pulling my raincoat on over my T-shirt, went outside to get the newspapers. The driveway was cold and gritty under my bare feet. It was also empty.

My car! I suddenly realized. *They've got my freaking car!* I had forgotten that it was impounded. And remembering that fact made me feel even worse than I already did after seven grueling hours of waking nightmares. I was not, to put it nicely, in a good mood.

Trudging back into the house with the newspapers, I tried to focus my thoughts on what to do next. Should I just hide out in the house, reading books and eating potato chips, until Sergeant Lincoln called and said I could have my car back? Or should I rent an automobile and try to get on with my life. If you could call it a life. Maybe the best thing would be to catch a cab to the airport and fly off to Italy or Greece until the heat blew over. *Until the heat blew over?* I was starting to think like a criminal. Or, more precisely, a thug from a 1940s gangster movie. I decided to put off making any decisions until after I read the papers and had another cup of coffee.

There was nothing in either *The New York Times* or *Newsday* about my dead girl. (*My* dead girl? How possessive I was becoming!) Everything must have happened too late to make the morning editions. Or maybe the cops decided not to release any information to the press until after the family had been contacted.

There were, however, plenty of other local murder stories in the news to get me through the morning. On Monday a fashion model had been raped and strangled at a famous designer's forty-two room "get-away" in East Hampton. The next night a high school student from Bellmore was stabbed to death in the men's room of a popular comedy club. On Wednesday a young mother of two was shot during a bank robbery in Westbury, and later in the day an eighty-six-year-old woman was beaten to death at home by her own sixty-three-year-old son. Long Island had had a busy week.

I folded up the papers and put them in the recycling bin. Then I went into the bathroom, stripped off my nightshirt, and took the longest, hottest shower I could stand. I was getting dressed when the phone rang.

"Hello?" I said, gripping the receiver so hard my hand hurt.

"Hey, babe." Philly's voice was soothing and stimulating at the same time. Like a cup of hot tea with cinnamon. "I just wanted to see if you're all right. Bitch of a night, huh? I can't think of nothin' else. What happened after I split? What time did you get home?"

I gave her a quick synopsis of everything that took place after she left. "That Sergeant Lincoln is pretty nice," I added. "He drove me home about one-fifteen. But you won't believe *why* he drove me home—"

"'Cause they keepin' your car as evidence."

"How did you know that?"

"'Cause that's what Woodrow said would happen, and he knows all that kind of stuff. Told me to tell you not to worry, though. Said he can get you a real good deal on a used car and we can bring it out to you tomorrow. Simple as pie."

"You're kidding! I don't believe it! That's great, Philly. I really appreciate that. But does he really think I have to *buy* another car?"

"He says unless somebody confesses or they solve the case right away, they'll probably have to keep your car for a few months at least. Cost you a pile of pennies to rent somethin' for that long. 'Sides, honey, Woodrow says when you get your own car back, his business'll buy *this* one back from you. Pretty slick, huh?"

"God, that's great! I can't thank you enough, Philly. Please tell Woodrow how grateful I am. What kind of car is it and how much will it cost?"

"It's a Dodge Shadow. Old, but in real good shape. Some guy just traded it in on a new Chrysler a few days ago. Woodrow says he can get the new plates for you and everything, and you can have it for three grand. You got that much handy?"

"No problem. I'll have it ready for you tomorrow."

"Good. We'll be out to your house 'bout noon. Gotta go," she said. "I'm not allowed to make personal calls. If my supervisor catches me on this phone she'll fry my ass in lard and serve it to the old folks for lunch."

She hung up before I could say anything more. I placed my receiver back in its cradle and silently cursed Philly's job—the dirty and depressing job she had worked at so conscientiously, and so good-naturedly, since she was nineteen years old. The job where—even as a woman with a spotless fifteen-year employment record—she was not allowed to make a personal phone call. More than ever, I was determined to help Philly become a good enough reader to get into a better line of work.

As soon as I took my hand off the phone it rang again. I jumped about a foot off the floor, then sat down on the bed to answer it.

"Mrs. March?" said the smooth, deep voice on the other end. "This is Detective Sergeant Lincoln."

"Oh, hi."

"Hi yourself," he said. I could imagine his freckles colliding in the creases around his smile. "I called to see if you could come into the office this afternoon. Would that be possible? Got a few more questions for you."

"Well, I guess it would be possible. I mean, I don't have any *plans* or anything. But I don't have a *car*, either, so it wouldn't be easy."

"You could call a cab."

"Will the Police Department pick up the tab?"

"No, we don't have funds for expenses like that. If you're really hard up, though, I'd be willing to help you out personally."

"Forget it," I said, annoyed with his patronizing attitude. "I can handle it. And I have to get to the bank anyway. What time do you want me to come?"

"Is three o'clock okay?

"Your wish is my command," I said with just a dash of salt. "Where's your office?"

"I'm at headquarters on Franklin Avenue in Mineola." He gave me the address and told me not to worry about finding the place. "Most cabbies know where we are," he said, with a nearly audible smile.

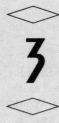

3

Franklin Avenue in the Garden City/Mineola area is often referred to as Long Island's Fifth Avenue. That's partly because the Long Island branch of Saks Fifth Avenue is enthroned there—along with Bloomingdale's, Lord & Taylor, and several specialty and designer shops—and partly because the pretty, tree-lined street offers good restaurants and nice office buildings to match its upscale shopping. I had spent a lot of time in the area before, but I had never noticed that the enormous tan brick building right next door to Saks was Nassau County Police Headquarters. I had always gone there looking for clothes, not cops.

The cab dropped me off right across the street from the main entrance, so I was treated to a full frontal view of the establishment. It looked like a huge hospital or high school. The flat manicured lawn stretching from the sidewalk to the face of the two-story structure was festooned with several fir trees, a few park benches, a tall flagpole complete with American flag, a big brass sign, and a cement walkway with metal handrails which bisected the lawn into symmetrical halves and led straight to the front steps. I crossed the street in the middle of the block, walked quickly up the center path, and entered the building.

Two uniformed officers were stationed in a large, glass-enclosed cubicle just inside the front door. One of them, a stocky man with slick black hair, asked if he could help me and I told him I was there to see Detective Sergeant Lincoln. As I spoke to him I found myself staring at the glass between us and wondering if it was bulletproof. The officer directed me to a phone painted with a wide red stripe hanging near the elevators, telling me to pick up the striped receiver and dial extension 78. I did as I was told.

"Detective Tupper, Homicide," a gruff voice answered.

"I, uh, I'm here to see Sergeant Lincoln," I stammered, feeling like a criminal for merely seeking entry to that decidedly male bastion of law enforcement. I had to remind myself that I had been *asked* to come here and that I hadn't done anything wrong even if they thought I had. "I'm downstairs in the lobby," I added unnecessarily.

"Do you have a name?" the gruff detective wanted to know.

"Oh, yeah!" I giggled, embarrassed at my omission. "It's Annie. Annie March."

"Hang on a minute," he ordered, clicking me on hold.

I sighed, wishing I was testing new lipstick colors and trying on sweaters in Saks instead of standing in the middle of Nassau County Police Headquarters, feeling awkward and out of place, holding a weird, red-striped phone receiver to my ear, wondering what the hell was going to happen to me next. I made a fervent promise to myself to never, ever leave my car trunk unlocked again.

"Okay, Annie March," Detective Tupper suddenly spit into my ear. "Stand by. I'm coming down to get you." He hung up before I could reply.

I stood by the elevators and the phone for a couple of minutes but nothing happened, so I strolled a few yards down the deserted hall, snooping around. I checked out a small exhibition case full of ancient police artifacts—old badges, a set of old handcuffs, an antique musket—and examined a large, prominent wall display of over a hundred wooden shield-shaped plaques. Each plaque featured a photo of a single policeman or policewoman and had a brass nameplate underneath. A larger brass plate was inscribed with the words: *In memory of the brave men and women who made the supreme sacrifice in the line of duty.* Directly beneath this display—as if in mockery—sat a metal rack full of gun magazines.

I sat down on the wooden bench next to the magazines, picked up a copy of *American Handgunner* and flipped through it. Lots of pictures of guns, bullets, and dead animals. I found it repulsive and quickly stuffed it back in the rack. I don't know a thing about guns. As far as I'm concerned, Smith & Wesson could be the name of a new salad oil. The only thing I know is that one of those guns killed my beloved Sam, and that I hate the horrible things as much as it is possible to hate anything in this life.

A beefy, sandy-haired man wearing a tan suit and a green tie approached me from the long hall to my left. "Are you Mrs. March?" he asked. I nodded, and when he stuck his hand out to shake mine, he bent toward me in an almost courtly fashion. "I'm Detective Nat Tupper."

I smiled and stood up. "It's nice to meet you," I said, although I wasn't sure it was.

"Come with me," he said, turning to head back up the long, empty hallway he had just walked down. "I'll take you upstairs to the Death Chamber."

"Death Chamber?"

"Our little nickname for the Homicide Department." He chuckled with pride.

"Oh," I said, unamused. I didn't think the poor girl from my trunk would have been amused, either.

Detective Tupper and I strolled to the end of the hall. He was in no hurry to get anywhere. He shuffled along in a sort of bow-legged squat, as if he had a load of gravel in his shorts. And as he lead the way up the wide staircase, I realized that, from the back, he also *looked* as if he had a load of gravel in his shorts.

"Is it always so quiet here?" I asked. "I mean, I've hardly seen any people, or anything."

"Everybody's working," he said, as if that explained everything.

When we reached the second floor I looked up and down the long wide hall, but I didn't see another soul. The brown linoleum floor gleamed like a wet highway. All of the doors on both sides of the hall were closed. Tupper waddled over to one marked 573 and put his hand on the knob.

"This is it," he said, waiting for me to reach his side. "There's no name on the door, so if any crazies come looking for us, they won't be able to find us." He opened the door, gave a little bow, and motioned me inside.

We entered a large room full of desks and people. There were six or seven men there, all wearing long-sleeved shirts and ties, and all acting busy in a leisurely sort of way. Some were talking on the phone, two were standing in a corner arguing about something, one was rifling through a file cabinet, one was eating a sandwich. A pretty, middle-aged woman with burgundy hair (Clairol's Loving Care would be my guess) sat at a desk right by the door and smiled at me as I walked in.

"You're here to see Eddie, right?" she asked.

"Right," I said, smiling back at her. Detective Tupper, suddenly in a hurry, pushed by me and made his way back to his own desk. As he passed by one of the men on the phone, he tapped him on the shoulder. Sergeant Lincoln turned around, looked in my direction and, still talking into the receiver, gave me a nod. He held one finger up in the air to let me know he'd be with me in a minute.

There didn't seem to be any place for me to sit, so I just stood there looking around at the old office furniture, avocado green carpeting, and wood-paneled walls. I felt self-conscious and I wasn't sure why. Maybe it was because I was surrounded by homicide detectives and they were all looking at me as if I'd be fun to finger-print.

"Sorry to keep you waiting, Annie," Sergeant Lincoln said, materializing at my side a few minutes later. "Do you mind if I call you Annie?"

"Not at all. Do you mind if I call you Mr. Ed?"

He let out a hearty laugh, which told me one of two things: either he was old enough to remember the early sixties television series about a talking horse, or he was prosperous enough to afford cable TV. I hoped it was both, because I was starting to find the tall, freckle-faced sergeant *very* attractive.

And I couldn't have been more shocked at myself if

I'd sprouted antlers and turned blue. Eddie was the first man I had looked at twice since Sam was killed. My sexuality had died with my husband. I hadn't even *thought* about sex. I had no idea why the amorous side of my nature was suddenly coming back to life after all this time, but I had no difficulty recognizing the symptoms: a flushed feeling around my face and neck, wobbly knees, heart palpitations, and a spiraling sensation in the pit of my stomach. I stared at my shoes and hoped my throbbing new infatuation wasn't noticeable.

"Thanks for coming," Eddie said. "I have a few things I want to talk to you about, but the boss wants to meet you first. He has some questions for you, too. His office is right down here." He turned and led the way down a narrow, uncarpeted walkway to an open office door. I followed him obediently.

Behind a small wooden desk positioned in the center of the tiny private office sat a trim, clean-looking man with wavy gray hair and enormous blue eyes. When he stood up to greet me I saw that he was of medium height and in great physical shape. He introduced himself as Detective Lieutenant Shawn O'Donnell. Then he asked me to sit down in the brown leather side chair against the wall and to the left of the door, which he closed as soon as Eddie left.

"I understand you had quite a night last night," he said, sitting back down behind his desk.

"That's a bold understatement," I said with a hefty sigh.

"I have here a copy of all the information you gave to Sergeant Lincoln at the scene, including everything you told him about your own life history." He held up several typed sheets of paper. "Have you thought of anything you forgot to tell us? Are there any details you could add?"

"If you're talking about my life history, I could give you volumes. Lots of pictures, too."

He didn't crack a smile. "No, I mean about the crime."

"I told Sergeant Lincoln everything I know."

"You and a friend, one Philomena Tripp, discovered the body in the trunk of your car at approximately 9:05 P.M. last night, is that right?"

"Right."

"And you have no idea how the body got there?"

"None."

"You notified the Hempstead Police immediately?"

"Yes, we did. My car was parked in the library lot right next door. As soon as we found the body, Philomena and I ran over to the station to report it."

"It says here that you attended the Paul D. Schreiber High School in Port Washington from 1968 to 1970. Is that correct?"

"Yes . . ." It was a *very* leading question, but what on earth was it leading to? Unfortunately, I didn't have to wait long to find out.

"So tell me, Mrs. March," said Lieutenant O'Donnell, taking aim at my face with his cold blue gaze, "how well did you know the victim?"

I was stunned. So much adrenaline was suddenly released in my bloodstream that I felt almost drunk. "What are you talking about?" I said, moving my mouth and tongue with difficulty. "I didn't know her at all. I never saw her before in my life!"

"Does the name Ben Masterson mean anything to you?"

"What? Who?" I was starting to get dizzy.

"Ben Masterson," he repeated. "Don't tell me you don't know who he is. I would find that very hard to believe."

"Well, I *don't* know who he is!" I insisted, working to regain my equilibrium. I was determined not to fall apart. If O'Donnell was going to challenge me in such an abrupt and hostile manner, I wanted to meet that challenge head-on. I took a deep breath, sat up straighter in my chair, and glared at him. "Would you mind telling me what this is all about? What makes you think I knew the victim? And who the hell is Ben Masterson?"

The lieutenant softened a bit. "You don't remember the name?"

"No, I don't. Why should I?"

"Because you and Ben Masterson were high school classmates."

I stopped breathing for a moment and searched frantically for a face to put with the name. I drew a complete blank. "I don't remember him at all," I finally said. "You're sure we went to school together?"

"Quite sure. He remembers you very well."

"*He* remembers *me*?" Panic started nipping at my ankles like a mean little dog. "Well, who is he, anyway? And what does he have to do with the dead girl in my trunk?"

"She was his half sister."

"Oh," I said, lowering my gaze to the ugly green carpet. My insides were twisted in tight knots of confusion, anger, and sadness. I felt sympathy for the victim and her family, and also worry about my own precarious position in the crazy unfolding scheme of things. "So you found out who she was," I said, bracing myself for the onslaught of more unwanted information.

"Her name was Jane Camille Masterson," Lieutenant O'Donnell revealed in a humdrum tone of voice, as if he were telling me something I already knew. "She was twenty-six years old, and she lived out at the Masterson estate in Sands Point, where she was born."

"Do you know when or where she was killed?"

"I can't discuss information relating directly to the case."

"Was she raped?"

"I can't answer that, either. I can only tell you what we've already told the press."

"Well, then, how did you identify her so fast? Had she been reported missing?"

"No, her half brother thought she was probably out on a date last night, and her mother didn't even know she was gone."

"So how. . . ?"

"That was the easy part," he said, becoming a bit more animated. "One of the charms on the bracelet she was wearing was a gold dog tag with her name, address, and phone number on it. We called the number, spoke to Ben Masterson, and he went immediately to the morgue to identify the body. Like taking candy from a baby."

I found the lieutenant's use of that particular cliché distasteful, but I didn't say a word. Another time-worn expression flashed through my mind and helped me control my behavior: never bite the hand that has the power to put you in the slammer.

There was a sharp knock, and Eddie opened the office door just enough to stick in his head. "Could I talk to you a minute, boss? Something's come up."

"Excuse me, Mrs. March." Lieutenant O'Donnell

got up from his chair and walked to the door. "I'll be back in a minute," he said, as if he actually thought I would miss him while he was gone. Leaving the door slightly ajar, he joined Eddie in the outer office, and a few seconds later, when I snuck a peek through the crack and down the hall, I saw them go into a room across the way.

I let out a muffled groan, leaned my head back against the wall and closed my eyes. *Ben Masterson, Ben Masterson. Was he the overbearing redheaded kid who sat next to me in Spanish? No, that guy's name was Ted something. Maybe he was the shy, skinny one in History who kept staring at me while he tapped his foot and picked his pimples. Or the hunk from my homeroom who ate paper and pencil erasers. . .*

"Sounds pretty messy," said a man's voice from down the narrow hallway. "Did she die immediately?"

"Yep," came the reply. The slow footfalls of two officers were moving toward O'Donnell's office, their voices becoming clearer with each step.

"Was she raped?" asked the first man.

"Is the ocean wet?"

"What about the crap they found wadded up in the bottom of the garbage bag?" The men stood still for a moment and there was a shuffle of paper, like pages flipping. My ears pricked: garbage bag?

"Just clothes. A big pink T-shirt, pair of gray sweatpants, white socks, and pink lace panties. No bra and no shoes. Strange thing is, except for the socks, each piece of clothing was cut apart in two or three places. With a big pair of scissors, or something."

I knew from things Eddie had said at the scene that the two men were talking about Jane Camille Masterson's clothes. I thought of sticking my head through the door to let them know I was there, but quickly decided against it. I figured I'd better eavesdrop instead, and use the opportunity to learn as much as I could about the murder—especially since it was beginning to look like they might try to pin it on me!

"How's about location? Any idea where she was popped?" The footsteps were coming closer again.

"Well, they found lots of debris in her hair and on her clothes—sand, humus, manure, moss, mica flecks—so it looks like she was either raped, or killed, or both, outside somewhere. On the ground. The knees of her sweatpants were embedded with dirt."

"She was probably praying."

"Or begging."

I nearly leapt from my chair as a loud knock sounded and the door flew open at the same time. The officers were clearly surprised to see the door give way, and to find me half-out of my seat, staring at them in shock.

"Oh," said one of the officers, "I thought I'd find Link—Sergeant Lincoln in here." I saw that he held a sheaf of papers in his hand.

"Oh, he's—Or, well. . . he'll be right back. They've just stepped out for a minute."

"Fine," the officer said, "I'll find him later. Thanks."

He turned to join his colleague in the hallway, then looked back at me and smiled. "Sorry if I startled you," he said, and left, shutting the door firmly behind him.

I was amazed. By just keeping my mouth shut and staying put, I had learned much of what O'Donnell refused to tell me about the case, and more. For some reason, this made me feel better. Like a cat dining on a canary. With a welcome surge of self-confidence, my composure returned. I chuckled softly and hummed a few bars of the theme from *The Pink Panther*.

∘ ∘ ∘

"Sorry to keep you waiting, Mrs. March," O'Donnell said as he marched back into his office a good ten minutes later. "And now I'm afraid I'm going to have to cut our interview short. Another appointment."

"That's too bad," I said. "I was hoping to get this over with." Frowning on the outside, grinning on the inside.

"Sergeant Lincoln will take up where I left off."

"Fine," I replied. Pouting on the outside, panting on the inside. What was happening to me? At the mere mention of Eddie's name my body became a hormone factory.

"I'll want to talk to you again soon," O'Donnell added, "and also with your friend Philomena Tripp. I'll be in touch." He grabbed his suit jacket from the hook behind the door and walked briskly away.

Eddie appeared in the doorway as soon as Lieutenant O'Donnell was gone. "Come on out to the bullpen, Annie. We can sit at my desk and talk."

I followed him eagerly into the large room. He pulled a chair from behind an empty desk, pushed it over next to his, and I sat down. "I don't believe what's happening!" I said as soon as he was seated in his own chair. "I never laid eyes on Jane Camille Masterson until I opened my trunk last night. I couldn't pick Ben Masterson out of a lineup even if every other fellow in the line looked just like Woody Woodpecker. And I've never, ever fired a gun in my life! How could O'Donnell think, even for a moment, that I had anything to do with this murder?"

"He *has* to think the worst of everybody. That's his job."

"And what do *you* think? Have you got a cute jail cell picked out for me already? Something in pink would be nice."

He smiled, and the way he looked at me, I wanted to curl up like a cat on his lap for eternity, or at least until next Sunday. "You can relax with me, Annie," he said. "I know you didn't do it."

"Well, it's nice to know I have at least one friend around here."

"And your list of friends will grow, I'm sure, as more and more details about the crime come to light." Eddie put his hands behind his head, leaned back in his chair and stretched his long legs out to the side of the desk. The sight of him in such a lazy, intimate, near-prone position made my flesh ripple. I wondered if he would look that splendid after making love.

"So, are there any more details you could give me?" he asked. "Have you thought of anything—any little thing at all—you forgot to report last night?"

"No. There's really nothing I could add, unless you want some more information about my personal life." *Such as what kind of wine I like, which restaurants I prefer, and what kind of music puts me in the mood.*

"What about Ben Masterson?"

"I don't remember him at all. The name doesn't even ring a bell."

"You don't remember anything about the family either?"

"Nope."

"And I guess you never heard of Jane Camille Masterson."

"Not until Lieutenant O'Donnell told me who she was."

"Doesn't look like there's much point in going on with this," he said, sitting up straight in his chair. "Wait here a second. I want to see if any new reports have come in from the Medical Examiner's office." He stood up and sauntered over to a desk on the far side of the room.

While Eddie was gone I studied the top of *his* desk, looking for clues to his personal side. Everything was neat and orderly. I liked that. Papers were stacked in careful piles; all pencils and pens were contained in a large red coffee mug. There were a few doodles on his blotter—cartoon faces and crazy-looking cars.

There was also a carefully printed list of notes in the lower margin of the blotter: *TOD*, it said. Tod? I turned slightly in my chair and looked again. *TOD 7-8* P.M.. A time. Time of death! Between 7 and 8 P.M.! These were notes about the murder—well, *a* murder. Could it be · mine? (I caught myself being possessive again.)

I strained to see the next couple of lines: *No slug. 9mm or .357?* Well, I'd seen enough TV cop shows to know the numbers referred to calibers of guns, and that "no slug" meant no bullet had yet been found. *Entry front-upper chest. Close rg. Exit lower spine. On her knees?* So it was a her, and this was definitely the path of the bullet, at close range. Sounded just like the wound I'd seen the night before. And the next few words on the blotter—*sand, moss, manure, mica*—made me certain that the notes pertained to the Jane Masterson murder. I read the whole list over again quickly, then sat back in my chair trying to appear as nonchalant—and as innocent—as possible.

Looking around for Eddie, I saw him standing on the opposite of the room, talking to one of the officers I had seen in O'Donnell's office. He showed no sign of immediately returning to his desk, so I took the opportunity to snoop around a bit more. A framed photo sat on top of a stack of papers, but it was turned away from me so I couldn't see what the picture was. I leaned against the side of the desk, casually stretched out my arm and nudged the photo with my finger until it was facing me.

My romantic flights of fancy about Eddie fell to earth with a thud. There, in the very center of the photo, sitting between two adorable freckle-faced kids, was an uncommonly beautiful woman with long brown hair, big blue eyes, and the deepest dimples you ever saw. And revealed in the low V-neck of her cream-colored silk blouse was the deepest cleavage you ever saw. It was enough to send any reasonably attractive woman with normal-sized breasts running for cover. In the interest of self-torture I stared at the photo for a few seconds and then quickly flicked it back to its original position.

Serves you right, I said to myself. *Getting a crush on a cop, for God's sake! How dopey can you be?*

Infinitely dopey, as it turned out. As soon as Eddie returned to his desk and sat down, I blurted out, "So, how's the wife and kids?" Right then I made the difficult but obviously necessary decision to have my mouth surgically removed.

"Oh," he said, "you must have seen the photo."

"Yeah," I admitted, staring at the carpet in shame. I wondered what cruel astrological or genetic joke had determined that I would be tongue-tied when I had something valid to say, and a blathering idiot the rest of the time.

"It's an old picture," Eddie said. "Taken about six years ago." He picked up the photo and looked at it. "Kevin's twelve now," he said, turning the photo toward me and pointing to the boy, "and Annette is fifteen. Claudine took both of them to live with her parents in Indiana for a while. I haven't seen them in over a month."

"That's too bad."

"Right," he said, putting the picture back down on the desk. "Just one of the hazards of this job. Around here marriages get killed as often as people."

"Is yours dead?" I asked, trying not to look *too* hopeful.

"Just wounded. They're coming home next week. We're gonna sew it up and see if it'll heal."

"Good luck," I said, surprised to discover that I really meant it. I liked Eddie a lot and wished him well in spite of my budding, but obviously doomed, desire.

"Thanks," he replied, seeming embarrassed. "Getting back to the case at hand," he said quickly, "I thought you should know that the Masterson funeral is going to be at ten o'clock on Monday morning. You might want to go. They're having it at St. Peter's in Port Washington. Do you know where that is?"

"Yeah. I went to high school near there, remember?"

"Right." He smiled. "Then maybe I'll see you at the funeral. For now, I think we're all finished here. Do you want me to call you a taxi?"

"No, thanks. I've got some shopping to do in the area. I'll get my own cab."

We said our good-byes and shook hands warmly. Then I hurried out of the building and darted next door to Saks, heading straight for the lingerie department. I picked out the prettiest black lace push-up bra I could find and went into the dressing room to try it on. It didn't give me Claudine-sized contours, but it *did* make me feel more womanly. And stronger, in a strange kind of way.

As I stood in line at the cash register to make my purchase, I wondered if they let you wear black lace in prison.

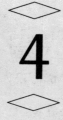

4

The first thing I did when I got home, before taking off my jacket or sunglasses, was go into my office, climb up on the desk chair, and take my high school yearbook down from the top shelf of the bookcase. I cracked the big blue book open to the index in the back, and went down the list of names in the M section. Macklin, Mafflehead, Mallory, Marlowe. There it was: Masterson, Benjamin Ramsey, pages 63 and 104.

Page 63 was part of the Basketball section. I found the name in one of the captions under the small black and white photos of the team in action, but the face wasn't visible in the picture. I quickly flipped to page 104. The Senior portrait section. And there *he* was. Benjamin Ramsey Masterson, a nice-looking, dusty-haired kid, wearing the required white shirt, tie, and dark jacket, casually aiming a cocky smile at the camera. I didn't recognize him. The copy under the photo said: *Basketball: 2, 3, 4; Soccer: 3, 4; History Club; Drama . . . He will grab the future in both hands and squeeze hard.*

I removed my sunglasses and took a closer look at the picture. A memory stirred and fluttered in the back of my brain. And then suddenly, like a homing pigeon, it flapped to the forefront. *Oh, yeah! That guy!* I used to flirt with him in English class. He sat right behind me. I thought he was funny and handsome, but I was going steady with Mitch Campbell at the time, so I never really got to know him or spend any time with him. We didn't hang out in the same crowd.

Ben had autographed his photo and also written a message to me in the top margin of the page: *To the prettiest Senior girl of all . . . I like to make you laugh, and I love to watch you walk. Stay as sweet (and sexy) as you are . . . Ben.*

I stared at his face for a few moments, trying to imagine what he would look like now, twenty-six years later. Then I turned to page 98, to my own graduation photo, to recall what I looked like twenty-six years ago. My name was Anne Hopkins then, but—thanks to a slight Southern accent left over from my Georgia birth and early upbringing—everybody called me Dixie. I was pretty cute, if I do say so myself. Short, curly dark hair, big dark eyes, bright smile. *She will laugh her way through life*, it said under my photo. Ha! Considering everything that had happened to me in the last five years, I found that prediction laughable.

I closed the yearbook and ventured into the kitchen to see what I could find for dinner. The refrigerator was pretty empty, but I managed to scrounge up the ingredients for a cheese and onion omelet and a green salad. I opened a bottle of dry white wine and drank two glasses while I prepared the meal.

When I sat down to eat I put on the TV as usual, but I couldn't pay attention. I kept thinking about Eddie

Lincoln, how attracted to him I was, and how odd it was for me to be attracted to *anybody*. I had come to accept celibacy as a natural, even preferable way of life. For five long years my libido had been in hibernation. And now, suddenly, it was completely awake and standing tall on its hind legs like a grizzly.

I wondered about this for a while, finally coming to the conclusion that my raging hormonal condition probably had as much to do with the death of the Masterson girl as with the desirability of Eddie Lincoln. Seeing her dead body in the trunk of my car had shocked me to the core, blasted me out of my own personal limbo. To put it tritely, coming face to face with death had heightened my desire to live. I wanted to eat, drink, be merry, and have sex before it was too late.

So I ate my dinner, drank the rest of the wine, and went to bed early, hoping I'd be merry and have sex in my dreams.

I don't know whether I fell asleep or passed out. It was probably the latter, considering the fact that I had consumed a whole bottle of wine. Whatever the case, I slept soundly through the night. I didn't have any dreams that I remember, but I awoke feeling as if I'd survived a few nightmares.

I took a shower and washed my hair, then blew it dry into a wanton frenzy. I put on a pair of blue jeans, a black T-shirt, and some makeup, and went outside to get the papers.

Newsday had put the story on page 3, along with a recent photo of Jane Masterson at her beautiful best. She looked young, exuberant, very blonde, and very much alive. The article and photo filled up more than half a page, but it gave out very little hard-core information. *The New York Times* managed to disclose the same data in three tight paragraphs, which they printed on page 28 of Section B. I was very relieved to see that my name was not revealed in either account. *Newsday* dubbed me "an unnamed individual" and in *The Times* I was referred to as "a library patron." There was no mention of Philly at all.

After reading the rest of the newspapers and downing my usual two cups of coffee, I ate a bowl of cereal and swallowed a handful of vitamins with a glass of low-fat milk. Then I did what I always do when I have no place to go, and feel too wound up to read a book, work on a freelance assignment, plan a reading lesson, or play the piano: I cleaned the house.

Some people go on eating binges when they're anxious. Others sleep, chew their nails, or run around the block. I clean things.

I vacuumed all the carpets and floors, except for the one in Sam's studio. I brushed the couches and chairs to remove the cat hair. Ripping around my little house like a robot on speed, I dusted the furniture, Windexed the mirrors and piano keys, scrubbed the bathroom, and put clean sheets on my bed. I would have mopped the kitchen and bathroom floors, but it was getting close to noon and I knew Philly and Woodrow would be there soon. So I put the Windex, the Comet, and the Hoover away, and began searching through the cupboard and refrigerator for something I could pass off as lunch.

Three cans of tuna and two cans of beans later, I had prepared an acceptable tuna salad with slivered onions and mayonnaise and a weird kidney bean and chickpea concoction with scallions, capers, and balsamic vinegar. I toasted a loaf of garlic bread I found in the freezer and, since there was nothing in the house to drink besides milk, coffee, and wine—the mere smell of which I knew would make me puke—I made a big pitcher of iced tea. I didn't have any lemons, but I found a reasonably fresh orange in the back of the vegetable bin which I cut into eighths and arranged in a green glass candy dish for color. By the time the doorbell rang, lunch was on the table.

Philly was starving, so we sat down to lunch right away. While we were eating I gave Philly and Woodrow a quick rundown of what had happened at police headquarters. We didn't talk about it for long, though, because Woodrow was in a big hurry and he kept urging Philly to eat faster. Saturday was his busiest day, he said, and he had to get back to work. But what was really happening, I think, was that he was terrified of my cats and frantic to get out of the house. I cleared the dishes off the table, stacked them in the sink, and we all went outside to look at my new car.

"Ain't this the slickest little getabout you ever saw?" Philly asked me. "It looks a lot like my Sundance, but it's older and cuter."

"It's perfect," I said, and it was. Compact, clean, and in almost-new condition. Shiny black with a soft gray interior, and only 42,000 miles on it. "I can't thank you enough, Woodrow. You've really saved my life."

Woodrow was beaming with pride. He stood tall on my lawn, legs apart and folded arms resting on the paunch of his belly, grinning as if he'd just won the heavyweight championship. His thick black mustache stretched wide across his broad face, and his yellowish eyeballs rolled around in their sockets, recording every detail of the moment with conspicuous pleasure. He loosened his tie and wiped a few beads of sweat from his dark brown forehead with a clean white handkerchief. "Want to take her for a spin?" he asked me. He wasn't in such a hurry to get back to work anymore.

"You betcha," I said. "Let's buzz up to the golf course and back. Want to come, Philly?"

"Naw. It's too nice right here. I'm jest gonna sit on your grass in the sun and smell the spring." As if to prove her words, Philly plopped to the ground in one quick motion, like an insecure scoop of ice cream from a cone. She sat cross-legged on the grass, rested her elbows on her knees, propped her head in her hands, and inhaled deeply. In her dazzling yellow blouse and her baggy, bright purple pants, she looked like an overgrown pansy.

"We'll be back in a few minutes," I said, opening the car door and getting behind the wheel. Woodrow squeezed his large body into the passenger seat and struggled to fasten his seat belt. I turned the key, the little car came to life, and we whistled off down the street in style. Well, sort of in style. As much in style as a secondhand Dodge Shadow can be. And as much in style as *I* have ever felt the need to be. The car was comfortable, easy to operate, and everything worked, including the radio. What more could you want for three thousand bucks?

I looked at Woodrow and gave him a big smile. "Just me . . ." I sang, "and my shaa-aa-dow . . ."

He laughed and patted my shoulder. Then all at once he turned serious. "I sure am glad I could help you out, Annie," he said with an obvious catch in his throat. "I've been wanting to do something nice for you for a long time. You've done so much for Philly. She's like a brand new person. Learning to read has been the best thing that's ever happened to her." He sounded for a second like he might start crying. A forty-eight-year-old car dealer near tears because his thirty-four-year-old wife was learning how to read.

I was impressed. During tutor-training at Literacy Volunteers of America we learned that some husbands don't want their wives to become literate. It threatens their supremacy. They like it better when their women have to depend on them for everything. More than one woman has come to LVA for help, been given a tutor and made progress in her reading, only to find herself in divorce court, or—worse—abandoned without a penny. I had always known that Woodrow wasn't one of those kind of men, but I hadn't realized how dedicated to Philly he truly was, how much he cared about her education, advancement, and self-respect. From that moment on, I was a big Woodrow Tripp fan.

"Philly isn't the only one who's better off," I told him. "Teaching her to read has been one of the best things that ever happened to *me*. After Sam's death I felt like I didn't have any reason to live. I was really lost. But working with Philly gave me something important to strive for—a whole new purpose, not to mention a wonderful new friend."

"We're all blessed to have each other," he said simply. Then he patted me on the shoulder again.

We drove in silence for awhile—zipping down shady suburban streets and dodging squirrels in our little car-cocoon of affection and good will. The azaleas were in bloom, splashing the lawns on both sides of the pavement with patches of intense color. Deep red, tender baby pink, succulent tangerine. For those few glorious minutes I felt free, happy and—like the azaleas—vividly alive. When we came to the fence and gates of the golf club, I made a U-turn and headed for home.

❖   ❖   ❖

"I'm surprised you haven't heard from Lieutenant O'Donnell yet," I said to Philly as she and Woodrow were getting into her car to leave. "He said he was going to call you to come in for questioning."

"He can question me till the North Pole melts," she said in a huff, "and he still won't get no answers. All I know is I saw a dead girl in your car and it scared the shoestrings right outta my sneakers. And now I can't sleep at night."

"I'm sure he'll call you anyway. He doesn't seem like the type to leave any stones unturned."

"He can call all he wants. I'll even go in to see him if I have to. But I still won't be able to tell him squat."

"Of course not! We can't tell him what we don't know! Meanwhile," I added, "he probably thinks we're both in this together."

"Yeah, right!" Philly said. "We shot the poor thing, took off every stich she had on, put her body in the trunk, and went to a public library?"

"So we would have an alibi, of course."

"But the library's right smack next to the police station!"

"Sure is," I said, "but we could have thought that would make us look even *more* innocent."

"Okay . . . 'spose he *does* think we did it. What could he rightly think is the *reason* we did it?"

"That's easy," I said. "He probably figures we were motivated by jealousy. That I wanted to kill her because she was young and rich, and that you wanted her dead because she was a natural blond."

Woodrow burst out laughing and Philly slapped him on the arm. "Don't you be laughin' at me, old man!" she said, smiling. "What *you* gonna do when they send me off to the hoosegow? Who's gonna make you ribs and mashed potatoes? 'Member how skinny you were when you were single?"

We all laughed together for a few seconds and then Philly started up her car. "Better get you back to work, baby," she said to Woodrow. "With your appetite, you got to bring home *lots* of bacon."

"Wait a minute," I said as she prepared to pull out of the driveway. "What do you think we should do about our reading lessons? Should we find another place to meet?"

"Heck no, girl! We got a good thing goin' just like it is. I'm not gonna let myself get scared off by some dumb old murderer. Are you?"

"No way!" I insisted, wondering if I was telling the truth. Philly's use of the word *murderer* made me realize, for the first time, that *somebody* had actually killed Jane Masterson, and that he was still out there, roaming around, maybe looking for somebody else to kill. He might even know my BMW license plate number. I had been so busy worrying about how to prove my own innocence I had forgotten all about the guilty one—the actual killer. I felt a sudden chill.

"So we'll meet next Thursday, right?" Philly asked.

"Same time, same place," I said.

On Sunday mornings Rockville Centre is a melodious town. There are so many churches in the area that during the hours between nine and noon the air resonates with the near and distant sounds of bells and chimes. I woke up with my usual ex-churchgoer's sense of *Oh, boy! It's goof-off-and-be-selfish day!* combined with *Watch out! It's time-to-feel-guilty day!* I tried to concentrate on goofing off and being selfish.

I wallowed in my warm sheets thinking of all the nifty things I could do before sunset: go for a long walk at Jones Beach; drive to the nursery and buy a huge pile of impatiens to plant in the yard; stop by the fruit and vegetable store for fresh asparagus and giant artichokes; go to the bookstore to see if Sue Grafton's new mystery had come in yet; shoot over to the Roosevelt Field Mall to check out the new line of T-shirts at The Gap. Life is full of exciting possibilities when you've got a car.

Due to a recent weight gain of two pounds and an imagined loss of all muscle tissue, however, I decided to start the day off by going to the gym. I got out of bed, put on my exercise tights and top, and went through the rest of my morning caffeine and cosmetics ritual. I left the house as soon as I was ready, before I could change my mind. Before the thought of scrambled eggs and the Sunday papers could get the best of me.

My gym—a pink-carpeted, fake fern-decorated establishment for women only—was very crowded, as it always is in the spring, when the threat of bathing suit season drives Long Island females into a calisthenic and aerobic frenzy. I worked out on the Nautilus machines for awhile and then fought for a place on the floor for the low impact class. While the instructor screamed "Work it!" and Ray Charles sang "Hit the Road, Jack," I marched and bounced and lunged with the rest of the latex-bound ladies, as if my life and my thighs depended on it. Forty-five minutes later, I was out of breath, slick with sweat, and ready to go home for a nap. I had atoned for some of my sins, I figured, but it would have been easier to go to church.

On the way home I stopped at the grocery to stock up on staples—cat food and kitty litter—then I drove straight back to the house. All my grand plans to bring flowers, fresh vegetables, literature, new clothes, and nature walks into my life—or, more specifically, into that very *day*—had vanished along with my energy.

I took a shower, coated myself in body lotion and put on a white sweatshirt with my favorite old gray sweatpants. I picked up both big fat editions of the Sunday papers, lugged them into the bedroom, and put them and myself on the bed. Legs stretched out and torso propped up on pillows, I began looking through *The New York Times Magazine*. I started reading an article about water pollution, but my mind kept drifting and my head kept nodding. Finally, letting my arms drop down to my sides, I rested the still-open magazine on the lap of my gray sweatpants and closed my eyes. *Jane Camille Masterson was wearing gray sweatpants when she was killed*, I remember thinking right before I dozed off.

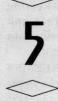

5

I went to Jane's funeral in my new black car and my new black-lace bra. I also wore a black knit dress, black stockings, and black alligator pumps. A high neckline concealed my cleavage and a low hemline covered my knees. I wanted to look like an innocent, respectable, and sympathetic mourner—not like the agitated, sex-crazed murder suspect I had become.

It was a half-hour drive from the south shore village of Rockville Centre to the north shore town of Port Washington, and I spent a large portion of it worrying about how I would express my sympathy to Jane's relatives at the funeral. What could I possibly say to her parents? *Please forgive me for finding your daughter's dead body in my car?* And Ben would be there, of course. What would I say to him? *Gee, I can't believe how long it's been! How have the years been treating you? Do you think I killed your half sister?* Nothing seemed appropriate.

I finally decided that I would follow one of the edicts of my Southern girlhood: I wouldn't speak unless I was spoken to. My prim and proper grandmothers would soar out of their graves with pride! I wondered if Eddie would be there. Maybe I could just stick with him and avoid the Masterson family altogether.

The morning rush hour was over, but that didn't keep another traffic jam from congealing on the ever-crowded Long Island Expressway. All the cars slowed down to a slug's pace, and all the drivers craned their necks over their steering wheels and peered ahead, looking for signs of an accident. Or, better yet, someone to blame and honk at. Luckily, my exit was the next one up, so I knew I wouldn't be stuck for long. But since I hadn't wanted to arrive at the funeral early and hadn't left myself any extra time, I also knew that even a slight delay would make me late.

I pulled into the church parking lot at twenty past ten and found a spot near the back of the building. Just a few cars were parked in the area. Wobbling uncomfortably on my three-inch heels—my Southern Methodist grandmothers thought high heels were the work of the Devil, and I believe they were right!—I hurried around the side of the ancient structure, up the front path to the church, and pulled open one of the weathered wood doors.

The grim atmosphere hit me in the face like a sheet of metal. The narrow church, with its arched ceiling and slender stained glass windows, was constructed of stone. The walls were stone and the floor was stone. The air was raw and damp. A center aisle led from the back of the church where I was standing straight down to the prominent, pall-draped coffin, which sat squarely in front of the altar.

I bypassed the dish of holy water stationed at the end of the aisle and began the walk down to the front where the people were sitting. The back two-thirds of the church was empty. High heels clicking noisily on the stone floor, I teetered my way past marble statues of Jesus, Mary, and John to an empty wooden pew behind the small group of mourners. There I sat down, put my purse on my lap, hugged my folded arms under my breasts, and shivered involuntarily.

"Give her eternal rest, dear Lord, and may your light shine on her forever," a deep male voice intoned. "And now, please turn to page forty and join with me in song."

The damp quiet was suddenly shattered by the harsh vibrations of too-loud organ music. The sound was so astonishing that I flinched and gasped aloud. The congregation stood up, and I did too, knocking my right shin against the padded kneeling rack—or hassock, I guess you'd call it—in the process. A few people started to sing, but their voices were completely swallowed up by the torturous wailings of the organ's enormous pipes.

After the soundless singing and earsplitting music subsided and the people were settled back in their seats, a young priest stood up to address the congregation. He had the blond hair and round, rosy cheeks of a cherub. After listening to his mechanical voice intone several routine, impersonal phrases, I decided that he hadn't known Jane Masterson from a hole in the ground—an unfortunate thought under the circumstances. I stopped listening to what the priest was saying and started looking around for Eddie.

He wasn't there. No friendly freckled face peeped, detective-style, from the shadows between the confessional booths. No tall lean figure in a trench coat lurked behind the candle nooks. And there wasn't one curly brown head to be found in the cluster of gray-haired and balding noggins displayed in front of me.

Most of the mourners appeared to be over the age of sixty. Where were Jane's friends? I wondered. Where were the girls she went to school with, the young men who took her to rock concerts and out to dinner? Where were her coworkers, her dancing partners, and her drinking pals?

I peered ahead and toward the right, looking for the Masterson family. There were only two people in the front pew. One seat in from the aisle sat a wiry, thin-shouldered woman with sparse beige hair and a tiny black straw hat. She held a white linen handkerchief to her face and quivered constantly, like a taut, just-plucked harp string.

Next to her, on the aisle, sat a large man with broad shoulders in a charcoal gray suit. A wavy mane of gray-streaked light brown hair hung over his collar and about three inches down his back. When he turned his head to the left for a moment, I saw that he had a dark brown mustache and a gold stud earring in his left ear. He didn't look anything like his yearbook photo, but I knew it was Ben. He was in the right age bracket and the right church pew.

Organ music suddenly swarmed through the air again and six men in dark blue suits appeared from nowhere. They hoisted up the coffin, balanced it high on their shoulders and walked down the aisle in my direction and toward the door. I stood with the rest of the congregation and said a silent personal prayer for Jane as she was spirited by.

Right behind the coffin came two priests, and behind them, Ben, with the beige-haired woman cling-ing desperately to his left arm. He was taller than I remembered and much brawnier. As he passed by my pew he looked straight into my eyes and winked.

Outside, in the crisp sunshine of the late May morning, the mourners milled around in a tight little group until the coffin was installed in the waiting hearse. Then they began walking, en masse, to the parking lot to get their cars. As I turned to follow them, a large hand grasped my shoulder from behind.

"It's good to see you again, Dixie," Ben said, moving around in front of me, blocking my passage. His sizable frame also blocked the sun, shrouding me completely in his cool shadow. "What's it been? Twenty-five years?"

"Twenty-six."

"Well, you're looking good as ever," he said, smiling. "You're coming to the cemetery aren't you?"

"I wasn't planning to," I admitted, looking up at his handsome, lightly tanned face. He had aged well and the mustache was an attractive addition. "Under the circumstances, I wasn't sure I'd be welcome."

"I want you to come," he insisted. "And I want you to come out to the house afterward. Other people are coming too. There's plenty to eat and drink. We can talk." His dark brown eyes urged me to comply. The sun burned behind him, illuminating the prickly wild ends of his flyaway long hair. It looked like little bolts of lightning were shooting out of his head.

That's when I made my momentous decision. Right then and there, standing in Ben Masterson's shadow outside the portal of St. Peter's, I devised my foolhardy plan: since Eddie wasn't there, I would play detective in his place. I would go out to the Masterson estate and learn everything I could about Jane's family and the other people she was close to. Maybe I would uncover something important—something that would put *me* in the clear. *And maybe the murderer himself will be there*, I speculated, feeling all brave and sleuthy inside. Those Nancy Drew books I had read as a kid were finally taking their toll on my sanity.

"Thanks for asking me," I said. "I'd be glad to come."

"Good." Ben smiled at me again. "Just follow the procession down Port Boulevard to Nassau Knolls Cemetery. I'll see you there." He strode quickly across the grass and got into the black limousine idling behind the hearse.

I hurried out to the parking lot, slipped behind the wheel of my Shadow, and searched madly through my purse for my car keys. I was buzzing with nervous energy. Excited and terrified at the same time.

Now, I'm not a *total* moron, so I *knew* it was a crazy scheme. The kind of dumb, stupid scheme they make dumb, stupid TV movies about. I knew I was putting myself at risk, biting off something I had no business even *trying* to chew. But I didn't care. I felt responsible for Jane, somehow, and I couldn't stomach the thought that her murder might go unsolved.

I also thought that if I could take an active role in finding Jane's killer it might help me live with the fact that my husband's murder had never been solved. Maybe it would ease the sickening sense of futility and helplessness that often overcame me, late at night, when the nightmares woke me up and left me wondering how God, or Fate, or whatever, could let a good man die while the evil one who killed him remained alive and free.

With a pounding heart full of fear, courage, anger, love, and revenge, I found my keys, turned on the ignition, and pulled into line with the other cars in the

funeral procession. In an effort to shake off my anxieties
and drown out the deafening silence of death, I shoved
a tape into the cassette deck and listened to Lyle
Lovett's sexy voice and humorous lyrics all the way to
the cemetery.

The graveside ceremony was quickly and efficiently
performed. The people were gathered, the prayers
were said and Jane Camille Masterson was thoroughly
interred before my three-inch heels had sunk completely into the soft spring earth. I walked with the others back to the roadway and got into my car while Ben
deposited the little woman with the black hat inside the
limousine. Then, much to my surprise, he slammed the
limo door and sprinted along the curb in my direction.
He pulled open the passenger door of my car and
quickly crunched his large body into the bucket seat
beside me.

"I'm riding with you," he said. "Don't want you to get
lost. Or change your mind and go home."

"What about your mother?"

"You mean my stepmother."

"Well, whoever she is," I said, "do you think she
ought to be left alone right now? She looks pretty distraught to me."

"She's not just distraught, she's sick. Cancer. And
she's been pumped so full of painkillers she won't even
know I'm gone."

"So Jane was her daughter?"

"Her one and only."

His casual tone disturbed me. I started up my car
and followed the automobile in front of me—a white
Mercedes with a license plate that said, ironically,
REBIRTH—down the narrow road to the cemetery

exit. With a rush of sadness, I wished Jane Masterson could experience a miraculous rebirth of her own. Then, sucking in a deep breath, I turned my attention to the murder inquiry at hand.

"It doesn't sound like you and your half sister were very close," I probed, taking my first baby step toward investigative brilliance.

"Hardly knew each other," he said, pulling a cigarette from the pack in his shirt pocket and lighting it with a blue Bic. "She was only one year old when I went off to Princeton. And once I went to college I hardly ever went back home. Take a left at the exit," he directed, "and keep going straight, past the church and all the way into Sands Point."

I moved into the stream of traffic heading north. The road was humming with expensive vehicles—the kind of imports the well-to-do inhabitants of Long Island's north shore won't leave home without. Well-dressed women drivers whizzed by me on the right, annoyed at my funereal speed, tearing off to urgent, life-or-death appointments with their manicurists.

"Why?" I asked.

"Why, what?"

"Why did you hardly ever go back home?"

"No reason to. My mother was dead. My step-mother, Bette, and I never liked each other. I thought she was a bore and she thought I was a brute. I liked my father all right, but he was never home. Always out of town on business. Germany one week, Japan the next. I didn't have a dog, so there wasn't any tail-wagging or face-licking to look forward to when I walked through the door."

"What about Jane?"

"Oh, she was okay, I guess, but she was just a little

kid. A lumpy, whiny, shy little kid. She wasn't any fun to be around. Nothing to go home for."

I wanted to ask more questions about Jane—what she was like when she grew up, what her interests and aspirations were—but I thought better of it. I didn't want to alert Ben to the fact that this was an interrogation, not a friendly, catch-up conversation between two old high school chums. "What did you do after college?" I asked instead.

"The usual stuff," he answered. "Went to law school. Harvard."

I smiled at the notion that Harvard Law School was the *usual* stuff. "And what came after Harvard?"

"Got married to a pretty young law student who decided she'd rather be Mrs. Masterson than Miss Representation." He raked his hair back from his forehead and fingered his gold stud earring. "Kate and I lived in Boston for a while and then moved to Aspen, Colorado where she became an unfulfilled housewife and I became the downest and dirtiest, not to mention the highest paid, divorce lawyer in town. Any more questions, counselor?" He looked at me with an unmistakable gleam—make that glint—in his eye.

He was on to me, I thought. Getting suspicious, or something. I shuddered, pushed down on the gas pedal a little harder and searched my brain for something diversionary to say. For once, my stupid blabbermouth came in handy. "Did you handle your own divorce?" I asked. "Sounds to me like you were headed for one."

"Whoa!" he squawked. "You really know how to hurt a guy." And when he turned his face toward mine I saw, with surprise, that he really *did* look hurt. A little angry, too.

"Sorry," I said, batting my eyes. I hoped my face was

properly flushed. "I didn't mean to upset you. I just wanted to save some time and get to the thick of things. Too many years have gone by for us to beat around the proverbial bush, right?"

Still unsettled and somewhat on the defensive, he hesitated. He gave me a squinty look and tugged on his earring again. Then, easily regaining his composure *and* the upper hand, he turned to me and said, "Whatever turns you on, babe."

I held my tongue for a while and waited for Ben to say something else. The white Mercedes was still in front of us, leading the way through the lush green shade of Sands Point's thickly treed acres. We were on Middle Neck Road, driving past the verdant lawns of the Sands Point Golf Club, when Ben nervously began beating out a drum roll on the dashboard with his fingers. "I could use a beer," he announced.

"Are we far from the house?" I asked.

"No. Just keep going straight. I'll tell you when to turn."

I looked around at the legendary landscape of huge houses on enormous pieces of property which had been known, during my high school years, as the "rich niche." Perry Como had lived here, I remembered, also Mafia boss Frank Costello and MGM mogul Nicholas Schenck. The Guggenheim estate was still out here somewhere, but it had been turned into some kind of public attraction. I wondered what Ben's father had done to earn *his* place in the Sands Point sun.

"I didn't see your father at the funeral today, Ben," I said, taking another tentative step in my inquisition. "Is he still alive?"

"No. He died a couple of years ago. Massive heart attack."

"I'm sorry to hear that. Were you and Jane the only children he had?" I asked, hoping to identify the heirs to the family fortune without being too obvious.

"Yeah," he said, letting out a spurt of bitter laughter. "The old man wasn't home enough to get either of his wives pregnant too often. Once apiece. That was his limit."

I suddenly saw Ben for what he was—a lonely, unloved rich kid who had grown up to be a lonely, unloved rich man. Not that I was feeling terribly sorry for him. With his cold and sarcastic slant on life, I imagined he was pretty good at withholding affection himself. And I was willing to bet that his wife—or ex-wife, if my guess was correct—could give him a good run for his money in the lonely department.

"Do you have any kids?" I asked.

"Not that I know of. After three miscarriages, Kate had her tubes tied. And if any of my other lady friends ever made me a father, they forgot to tell me about it." His offhand manner was contrived, I thought. Camouflage for intense feelings. "Take your next left," he said, "and take it slow. It's a tight corner."

I made the turn and fell in behind the REBIRTH license plate still winding along the road in front of me.

"You can follow the white Mercedes ahead," Ben said. "That's Dr. Stanwyck's car and he's going to the house. You can turn in behind him."

A wide cobblestone driveway with stone pillars eventually opened up in the long row of tall, thick fir trees on the right. As Ben had predicted, the white Mercedes turned into the passage and disappeared from view. I followed and caught sight of the car again on the serpentine private road which led to the Masterson mansion through well-tended borders of scarlet azaleas and purple rhododendrons. The car pulled to a stop at one edge of the circular cobblestone drive near the entrance to the house, and a middle-aged couple got out. Dr. and Mrs. Stanwyck, I presumed. There were two or three other cars parked in the area.

"Don't stop here," Ben instructed. "Keep on going around the side of the house. We'll go in the back door." He gestured ahead to a narrower, flower-banked roadway which took us around and behind the enormous residence, past the fenced-in tennis courts, past the cabana and swimming pool, and past the greenhouse and gardener's quarters. We parked where the road ended, at the far side of the main house by the attached four-car garage.

It wasn't until I got out of the car and took a good look around that I realized the full scope and beauty of the Masterson property. The wonderful old three-story home was built of gray stone, white stucco, and dark, walnut-colored wood which gleamed as if it had just been stained and polished. Several wood-railed balconies and outdoor walkways adorned the upper stories and an enormous veranda wrapped around the rear and one side of the ground floor. Rolling green lawns, towering shade trees, exquisitely landscaped terraces and patios embraced the house on each side. Flowers and shrubs bloomed everywhere.

And beyond it all, way out beyond the tennis courts, swimming pool, and greenhouse, stretched the grassy, private, pebble-beached coast of Manhasset Bay. The sweeping, unobstructed view was dazzling. You could see all the way across the flat silver sheet of salt water to the King's Point peninsula.

I wondered what it had been like growing up here, in this lap of loveless luxury. And as I turned to follow Ben down the slate path to the back door of the house, I imagined a chubby little golden-haired girl named Jane Camille playing by herself in the flower garden.

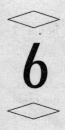

6

We entered the house through the kitchen, a window-lined room with white tiled walls and counters, stainless steel hardware and appliances, a huge butcher block worktable and a ceramic floor of tiny black and white hexagons. Bowls of fresh-cut flowers splashed color around the room—in the corners of the counters, under the wood-framed windows and glass-paned cupboards. Two fifty-something women in black and white uniforms stood on one side of the worktable arranging deviled eggs and finger sandwiches on gold-rimmed china platters.

"Hello, girls!" Ben called to them as we walked in. "Don't mind us. We're just passing through." He went straight to the refrigerator and opened it wide. He took out a bottle of imported beer and pried off the cap with an old-fashioned opener mounted on the wall nearby. Throwing his head back, he guzzled down half the bottle.

"Want one?" he asked me.

"Sure," I said, suddenly dying of thirst. I took the bottle he opened for me and followed him into the formal dining room.

A few people were standing around the long mahogany table in the center of the room. They were speaking in murmurs and heaping their plates with little crab cakes and mushroom crepes and apple walnut salad. There were baskets of warm rolls and croissants, a tray of bacon-wrapped chicken livers, and a big bowl of pasta topped with broccoli and sesame seeds. I wanted some of everything.

"You hungry?" Ben asked.

"You read my mind," I said.

"Well, just help yourself while I go upstairs and grab a pack of cigarettes, okay?"

"Fine."

Ben left the dining room and I decided to stand by the table, eat fast, and get it over with. After all, I wasn't there to stuff my face, but to conduct a murder investigation. I needed to talk to people and gather as much information as possible. I took a swig of my beer and popped a chicken liver in my mouth.

Before I could chew and swallow it, a stooped, white-haired old woman sidled over to me and wrapped her bony fingers around my wrist. "You can't budge a cook by his lover," she whispered. At least that's what it sounded like she said.

"What?" I asked, after one chomp on my chicken liver. Thinking she would whisper her words again, I leaned down and put my ear closer to her mouth.

"I said you can't judge a book by its cover!!" She screamed so loud that I jumped back and swallowed the chicken liver whole. Everyone in the room turned to look at us with startled expressions on their faces, and one of the maids dashed in from the kitchen nervously drying her hands on her apron.

"Now, now, Daisy," she said to the old woman, "what

do you want to make such a fuss for? There's nothing to shout about." The maid slipped her arm around the old woman's shoulders and began maneuvering her away from the table. "Come on out to the kitchen with me and I'll fix you a big glass of cherry soda."

The old woman's face lit up and her mouth curved into a beautiful smile. She fingered the organdy collar of her blue flowered dress and compliantly walked away with the maid. Just before she went through the door she turned back to me and called, "Don't forget what I told you!" Her ink-black eyes stared intently into mine for a few seconds and then she disappeared.

Astonished, I looked around at the other people standing in the dining room. They were all looking back at me, shrugging their shoulders, shaking their heads, and mumbling things like tsk, tsk and tut, tut.

"They ought to put that crazy old crow away," I heard somebody say. "She's an embarrassment."

"It's a shame," somebody else replied. "A real shame."

Just then Bette Masterson appeared in the dining room doorway looking very weary and wobbly. She held onto the hand-carved wood doorframe with both hands as her watery gray eyes circled the room. "I must apologize for my sister," she said in a shaky, high-pitched voice. "She's been under a lot of stress in the last few days. She's not herself." The woman looked so unsteady I thought she might lose her grip on the doorframe and fall face down on the beautifully polished parquet floor.

I knew a good opportunity when I saw one. I whisked across the room to Bette Masterson's side, placed one arm around her waist and the other beneath her elbow.

"You don't have to apologize for anything," I said,

encouraging her to shift her weight from the doorjamb onto me. "Your sister didn't do anything wrong. Now hold onto my arm and let me help you back to your seat."

She sighed heavily and allowed me to lead her away from the dining room. As we headed into the huge entrance hall, I took one last, longing glance over my shoulder at the mushroom crepes and crab cakes.

In the time it took me to navigate Mrs. Masterson across the ocean-sized blue Persian rug in the hall, all thoughts of food were driven from my mind. The poor woman trembled violently—a sure six points on the Richter Scale. Each step she took was an exercise in willpower and blind optimism.

Eventually we made it into the front parlor—a football field full of antique furniture and rugs, large vases of fresh flowers and numerous brocade couches and chairs. I led Mrs. Masterson to the couch nearest the entrance and helped her sit down. Finally settled and propped against a big red velvet arm cushion, she was still quaking.

"Thank you, dear," she said, looking up at me. Her wet gray eyes were full of pain. "It was kind of you to help me. What did you say your name was? My memory isn't what it used to be."

"We haven't been introduced yet, Mrs. Masterson," I said, sitting down next to her. "My name is Annie March."

"It's a pleasure to meet you, Annie," she said. Polite to the point of perfection. "My name is Bette. Please call me Bette." She patted my arm with a shaking, blue-veined hand. She wore an enormous emerald and diamond ring on one of her fingers. "Were you a friend of Jane's?" she asked. When she uttered her daughter's name a look of sheer horror shot across her wrinkled face.

"No. I'm a friend of Ben's. We went to high school together."

"Oh, that's nice." She gave me a shapeless smile.

"I'm so sorry about your daughter," I said, taking her hand in both of mine and stroking it softly. "It's a terrible, terrible tragedy." I looked at her thin shoulders and wondered how they would ever be able to bear such sorrow. Sam's murder had almost *killed* me, and I had been young and healthy as a horse.

"Yes . . ." she said, "terrible . . . tragedy . . ." Her eyes glazed over and she stared vacantly ahead, into the bleak, airless atmosphere of the harrowing days to come. Days upon endless days without her daughter.

"This is a wonderful house, Bette," I said, quickly changing the subject. "Have you lived here long?"

"What?" she muttered, stumbling back from the future to the present. "Oh . . . uhhh . . . Why, yes. Yes. I've lived here quite a while now. Almost thirty years. Ever since Ramsey and I were married."

Her eyes glazed over again and she left on another journey—this time into the past. "Ramsey and I met two years before we married, while I was studying music at Julliard. I was twenty-two. At that time I wanted to be a concert pianist and travel all over the world, but after I fell in love with Ramsey, I just wanted to be with him." She smiled at the memory.

I couldn't tell if it was a smile of rapture or remorse. I was too busy adding up the years, counting on my fingers I'm ashamed to say, trying to figure out how old Bette was. She was fifty-three or fifty-four, I calculated. Only ten years older than I was. What a shock! She looked more like seventy-five or eighty.

"Of course after we were married he was hardly ever home," Bette went on. "Always away on business. He bought me a beautiful piano," she said, gesturing toward the ebony grand dominating the far side of the room, "but after a while I stopped playing. What's the point of making music if there's nobody there to hear it?" She stopped talking for a few seconds and stared down at the once-talented hands now shaking involuntarily in her lap.

"It's hard to believe," Bette continued, "but I don't think Ramsey and I spent more than five or six days in a row together, from the day we married to the day he passed away."

"Does your sister live with you now?" I asked, changing the subject again, trying to keep the poor woman hopping over and between the deepest puddles of pain.

She nodded sadly. "Daisy moved in with me two years ago, right after Ramsey died. I would have taken her in long before that, but Ramsey wouldn't hear of it. He thought she would be a bad influence on Jane."

"Why?" I asked, glad to be getting back to the subject of Jane.

"Well, as you probably realized earlier, Daisy's not quite right in the head. Before I brought her to live with me, she was confined to an institution. Jane was a very impressionable girl and Ramsey didn't think it would be good for her to spend time around Daisy. Maybe he was right. Ever since the accident my sister's been terribly confused."

"The accident?" I wondered aloud.

She opened her mouth to speak, but before she could get a word out, Ben entered the living room and breezed over to us. I could tell from the frown on his face he wasn't too happy to find me sitting with his stepmother.

"I thought you were going to have lunch," he said to me.

"I was, but there was a slight disturbance and—"

"Your friend Annie is very nice, dear," Bette interrupted. "She helped me get comfortable here and we've been having a little talk."

"Well, *I'd* like to talk to her now, if you don't mind." His eyes dared her to object.

"Of course I don't mind, dear," Bette replied. "You two run along. I'll be fine right here on the couch."

Ben held his hand out to me and when I took it, he pulled me to my feet. "Let's go out on the porch," he said. "It's stuffy in here."

He marched me back through the hall and into the dining room, toward the French doors leading to the veranda. As we passed by the buffet, I retrieved the beer I had left sitting on the end of the table and took a big gulp. I hoped it would wash down the chicken liver that had rented a room in my midsection, somewhere between my larynx and my lungs.

Outside on the shady veranda, amidst the potted geraniums and giant ferns, a man and a woman were seated on wrought iron chairs with flowered cushions. I recognized the couple as the passengers of the white Mercedes with the REBIRTH license plate. They were sitting apart, on opposite sides of a glass-topped wrought iron table, sipping their drinks and staring wordlessly out at the horizon. A bottle of Chivas Regal sat on the table between them.

"Oh shit," Ben muttered under his breath when he saw them.

The man noticed us standing there, raised his glass

in greeting, and motioned us over to the table. "Hello, Ben," he said.

"Hi," Ben reluctantly replied.

"How's Bette doing?" the man asked. "Does she need anything?" His bloodshot blue eyes were swimming in grief. Or boozy self-pity.

"She's okay," Ben answered.

"If she recovers from this tragedy it'll be a miracle," the man said, rubbing the back of his neck with one hand and raising his glass to his lips with the other. The woman sitting with him said nothing. She shot an insolent glance in our direction and then quickly returned her gaze to the shoreline.

I remembered seeing these people at the funeral, but at first glance and from a distance, I had thought they were older than they now appeared to be. The man's somber suit, wire-rimmed glasses, and frizzy, platinum gray hair said late fifties, but his boyish, unlined face said early forties. I guessed the woman to be about thirty-five, but it was hard to judge. Most of her hair was hidden under a taupe-colored turban style hat, and she had the rigid bearing and taut, aristocratic facial features of a woman more advanced in age. She was impeccably dressed in a tailored navy blue suit and a taupe silk blouse.

"Who's your friend, Benjamin?" the woman asked, still staring straight ahead at the deserted beach.

"This is Annie March," he replied. "Better known as Dixie. We went to high school together."

"Glad to meet you, Annie," the man said, standing up and extending his hand for me to shake. "I'm Dr. Stanwyck. Niles Stanwyck. And this is my wife, Nina." He pointed his glass of scotch toward the tailored, turbaned woman who still hadn't bothered to turn her face in my direction.

"It's nice to meet you, Dr. Stanwyck," I said, ignoring the woman who was so blatantly ignoring me. "Are you Bette's doctor?"

"No!" he said, grimacing. He quickly removed his hand from mine and began rubbing the back of his neck again. His sad blue eyes darted from the floor, to the table, to the chair and back to the floor. "I was Jane's doctor," he mumbled.

Jane's doctor? I wondered what field of medicine he was in, and why Jane had needed him. I wanted to ask Dr. Stanwyck these questions, but I thought it would make me sound nosy and insensitive. I chose to wait and see if the information would be voluntarily revealed in the conversation.

I didn't have to wait long. "He was Jane's doctor, all right," Nina Stanwyck growled, suddenly lurching around in her chair and glaring at her husband. "He was Jane's own, personal Doctor Frankenstein!" She flashed a nasty, blood-red smile in my direction.

Niles Stanwyck's fragile composure cracked. "Shut up, you bitch!" he cried.

Everybody was quiet for a few seconds—just long enough for the air around us to grow mud-thick with tension. Then Ben stepped in to break the silence. "Jane had some cosmetic face and body work done," he explained to me. "Dr. Stanwyck was her plastic surgeon."

"Oh," I said. Not a very stunning response, but I was too uncomfortable to think straight. Niles and Nina were giving off some violent vibrations. Ben was still acting kind of hostile. I felt insecure and out of place—like a traditionally dressed, bonnet-topped Quaker woman in a room full of naked people.

Unable to think of anything to say, I used the time to

sneak my first careful, up-close look at Nina Stanwyck's face. She was obviously very drunk. And also very beautiful. Wide green eyes with thick dark lashes. Perfectly straight nose and prominent cheekbones. The rim of hair visible around the edge of her turban was the color of honey. She looked like Marlene Dietrich without all the feathers, flash, and sparkle.

I couldn't help wondering if her face had been designed by nature or by her husband.

Finally, my tongue came untied. "Would you excuse me please?" I said quickly. "I have to powder my nose." When in doubt, go to the bathroom. "Which way do I go?" I asked Ben.

"Up the main stairs, third door on the right."

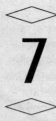

7

In the bathroom, I really *did* powder my nose. I put on some lipstick too. Then I left to carry out my *real* purpose for coming upstairs.

I went to look for Jane's room.

I like to snoop, but I'm not very good at it. I get too nervous. As I tiptoed down the Oriental carpet runner lining the long, wide hall, my heart was beating like a kettledrum in an echo chamber. My forehead broke out in a sweat and I was having trouble breathing. The anxiety began to melt away, however, once I became interested in the objects around me—especially the two large family portraits hanging side by side on the wall, each bathed in a golden glow from its own spotlight.

Both were oils, and both were painted by the same artist, somebody named Winterspoon. They were the same size and they were identically displayed in antique wood frames with gold nameplates. The one on the left pictured a family of three: a large, powerful-looking man with thick brown hair and bushy black eyebrows; a lovely young woman with peachy skin, dark brown eyes, and short auburn hair; and a boy of eight or nine with a dust-colored crewcut and a crooked smile. The gold plate under the portrait said: Ramsey Dodd Masterson, Ellen Grace Masterson, and Benjamin Ramsey Masterson.

The painting on the right pictured another family of three: a large powerful-looking man with thick gray hair and bushy black eyebrows; a thin, pretty woman with gray eyes and a silky light brown bob; and a girl of nine or ten with dark curls, a *very* pudgy face, and a slit for a smile. The gold plate underneath said: Ramsey Dodd Masterson, Bette Elaine Masterson, and Jane Camille Masterson.

I studied all of the faces in each of the portraits, trying to glean some truth, some knowledge, from the swirls of color on canvas. It was a wasted effort. The lifeless images stared back at me, flat and uncommunicative, revealing nothing. The only thing I learned was that young Jane Camille had been a chubby brunette instead of the delicate golden girl I had imagined. I left the mute Mastersons in spotlit suspension and crept on down the corridor.

The hall was long and wide enough to accommodate lots of furniture. There were tables, chairs, bookcases, and several wood and glass display cases. One of these cases held hundreds of hand-carved ivory figurines—ships, antelopes, birds, people. Elephants carved out of their own tusks. I wondered how many magnificent adult male elephants had been slaughtered to provide trinkets for the wealthy.

And how many magnificent young human females had been murdered to provide kicks for the sick.

I turned away from the trophy case and resumed my search for Jane's room. It didn't take me long to find it.

All the doors on each side of the hall were either wide open or slightly ajar. All but one.

It reminded me of the door to Sam's studio—the only door in my house that was always kept closed. I tip-toed up to it, took a deep breath, and carefully turned the hand-painted porcelain doorknob. Luckily, it wasn't locked. And I knew, the minute I looked inside, I had come to the right place. Everything about the room—the plush yellow carpet, the fluffy white bedspread splattered with purple violets, the elaborate CD player and speaker system—said *this* was a young woman's domain.

I slithered inside and quickly closed the door behind me. Then I froze there for a few seconds, with my high heels sinking deep into the thick carpet, shaking with dread and panting like a fat jogger. It wasn't just the fear of being discovered that made me so nervous. It was the thought that I was actually *there*, in *Jane's* room. The room where she had gotten dressed and brushed her hair and put on her makeup. The room in which she had lived and laughed and wept and slept and dreamed her dreams and planned her future. The room she would never set foot in again.

The sheer white curtains were drawn, but diffused sunlight still shimmered through the row of floor-to-ceiling windows on the far wall. In front of the windows and near the French doors leading to a balcony, sat a small round breakfast table surrounded by four purple and yellow flowered chintz chairs. A king-sized bed strewn with ruffled white and violet throw pillows dom-inated the room; opposite it were two large oak dressers and a beautiful antique dressing table with a matching wood-framed oval mirror.

But the desk and bookshelves to my immediate right

interested me the most. That's where I hoped to find out *who* Jane *was*. I hobbled over to the desk—my knees shaking and my heels continuing to get caught in yellow carpet fuzz.

It was organized and tidy, but I had no way of knowing if Jane, or the maid, had kept it that way. Pencils, pens, markers, a magnifying glass, and several pairs of scissors were contained in unique desk accessories—an assortment of small porcelain planters and clay flowerpots. A heavy piece of glass covered the work surface and weighted down the numerous magazine cutouts of plants and flowers—mostly irises—positioned underneath. A batch of trade paperbacks—all books about gardening—were propped between marble bookends on top of the desk.

Hardly breathing, I stared at the desk drawer for an eternity before I got up the nerve to open it. Finally, I looped my index finger through the circular brass handle and gently pulled it all the way out. There wasn't much inside. A blank note pad, some stationery, a small box of paper clips, and a large box of pushpins. A brown leather-bound Filofax was stuck way in the back, behind the stationery.

I snatched the leather book out of the drawer, unsnapped the closure tab and quickly turned through the daily calendar section to Thursday, May 14th—the day Jane was killed—to see what she had planned for that date. Nothing. Zilch. I flipped through the pages, going back in time, looking for interesting notations, but if that Filofax gave a true picture of Jane's activities, the last few months of her life had been *very* uneventful. I noticed several appointments with Dr. Stanwyck, a few trips to Manhattan, a couple of flower shows, but that was all.

With a fit of the jitters—but not a twinge of guilt—I ripped open the zipper of my shoulder bag and stuffed the book inside. Then I zipped the bag closed and hugged it to my body, all the while marveling that I had even had a chance to *find* the book, much less *steal* it. Surely the police had been there already, probing every nook and cranny, going over the room with a fine-tooth comb. Or had they? If they had discovered Jane's appointment book, wouldn't they have taken it with them back to Headquarters? Was it possible that I had been the first to discover it?

Too pressed for time to worry about questions I couldn't answer, I turned my attention to the low, wide bookshelves lining the wall to the right of Jane's desk. They were filled with magazines—hundreds and hundreds of fashion and beauty magazines. Month-by-month and year-by-year collections of *Glamour*, *Vogue*, *Elle*, *Cosmopolitan*, *Mademoiselle*, and *Vanity Fair*. The copies were arranged by title, in chronological order, with the latest issue of each magazine sitting on the surface of the uppermost shelf. There was an article of mine in the current *Cosmo*—a ridiculous fluff piece entitled "How to Turn Your Bedroom Into a Love Jungle" (get a tiger-striped bedspread, buy lots of plants, install a humidifier, etc.)—and I wondered, with a shudder, if Jane had read it.

An enormous bulletin board covered the entire wall above the bookshelves. And tacked to the cork with colorful plastic pushpins were dozens of photos of famous models. Cindy Crawford, Carol Alt, Claudia Schiffer, and all the others whose faces were familiar, but whose names I didn't know. Some of the photos were color and some were black and white. Some were head shots and some were full-figure pictures. Most had been cut from magazines, but some were glossy professional prints. A few of the glossies had been autographed.

In the lower right-hand corner of the bulletin board were several snapshots of Jane. I moved closer to the wall and studied them carefully. They were color prints, all taken on the beach, and it looked as if they were shot at the same time on the same day. Jane looked beautiful. And, from the way she was smiling, I would say she *felt* beautiful too.

She was wearing a black bikini and her windswept blond hair was as shiny as a swarm of sunbeams. Her body looked perfect—every bit as perfect as the bodies of the famous models tacked on the bulletin board around her. Whatever part Niles Stanwyck had played in the shaping of Jane's face and figure, he had done a good job.

But as I stood staring at those beautiful pictures of Jane, I couldn't help remembering how she had looked the first and last time I'd seen her—naked and bloody and heaped like garbage in a green plastic trash bag. Suddenly, I was sick to my stomach and consumed with rage. And bristling with renewed purpose. Somebody, somewhere, had turned this perfectly lovely young woman into the ugly, desecrated corpse in my car—and I intended to find out *who*.

Worried that I had been away too long, that Ben might come to look for me, I cracked the door open and peered out into the hall. It was empty. I slipped into the corridor, and closed the door behind me. Then I headed for the stairs, walking as fast as I could without running.

As I was making my mad dash down the hall I saw movement—a flash of white—in one of the open doors ahead. I slowed down a bit and looked into that room as I was walking by. Bette Masterson was lying down, still dressed, on her big four-poster bed, with some sort of compress on her forehead. A nurse in a white uniform was standing at the night table next to the bed, shaking capsules into her hand from a big brown bottle. I hurried away from the sorrowful sight and went to look for Ben.

I found him where I'd left him—on the veranda. But now the Stanwycks were gone and Ben was sitting down on a wicker couch at the end of the porch. He was partially hidden behind a bank of giant ferns.

"What took you so long?" he asked as I approached. "I was about to go hunting for you."

I doubted that. He looked too stoned to go hunting for anything—except, perhaps, another joint. His eyes were vague and his smile was even vaguer. A hint of marijuana smoke still lingered in the air.

Ignoring his question, I sat down next to him. "Where did the Stanwycks go?" I asked. "Back to Transylvania?"

He laughed. "Back to their home-sweet-home. They live just a few blocks from here." He took a Marlboro from the pack in his shirt pocket and lit up.

"Are they good friends of yours?"

"Nope. We never met until two months ago when I first came back from Aspen. Jane had them over for drinks a couple of times. They were *her* friends. Well, Niles was, anyway. She saw him almost every day— either for consultation or treatment or a quick lay on his office couch."

"Niles was Jane's lover?" I was shocked. The information I was gathering about Jane that day was *not* conforming to my mental picture of her. In my mind she had been a total innocent, tender and pure, struck down in her youth by a faceless force of evil. So much for my mind. Still, it was hard for me to imagine *any* woman having bags of silicone stuffed into her breasts, or globs of fat sucked out of her thighs, and then having an affair with the surgeon afterward.

"How do you know they were sleeping together?" I asked Ben. "Did Jane tell you herself?"

"Yeah. Said she was stuck on the guy and had been making it with him ever since her second nose job."

"She had *more* than one nose job?" The plot was thickening.

"Just two, I think."

"Do you know when she had her first one?"

"No."

"Does Nina know?"

"Know what? When Jane had her first nose job?"

"No!" I said, smiling. "Does she know that Jane and her husband were lovers?"

"Hey! What do I look like, a swami or something? I've got balls, but they sure as hell aren't crystal."

I giggled as if that was the funniest thing I ever heard in my life. I didn't want him getting suspicious again.

Ben turned his handsome face toward me and gave me a sexy, stoned smile. "I used to love to make you laugh," he said. "Sometimes I would spend my whole study period trying to think up jokes to spring on you in English class. Hell of a lot of good it did me. You were so hung up on Mitch Campbell, you didn't even know I existed." He took a deep drag on his cigarette and flicked some ashes on the floor. "But that was a long time ago. And now we're getting a second chance. Now that I'm divorced and your husband is dead."

My heart vaulted into my throat. "How did you know

that? Who told you about my husband? Was it Eddie, I mean Sergeant Lincoln?"

"He may have said something, but I already knew. Heard about it a year ago, after our 25th high school reunion. I didn't come in for the shindig, but an old friend of mine—remember Glen Busby?—he called me up after it was over and told me you were there. Said he danced with you and talked to you for a while. He said your husband had been murdered. That everybody at the party was talking about it."

"Oh . . . yes . . . Glen. I *did* talk to him for a few minutes. But I didn't realize—"

"What difference does it make who told me, anyway? The point is I *know*, and now you *know* I know, so we don't have to talk about it anymore, right? Your husband was killed, my sister's been killed, and that's just the way it goes in this fucked-up world. Nothin' we can do about it. What's dead is dead." He dropped his cigarette on the floor and ground it out with the heel of his black suede loafer. "And what's alive should be living it up." He gave me a suggestive wink. "In case you didn't know it, that means *us*, babe."

He was coming on strong. His dark eyes were driving into mine, demanding my complete attention, making silent but oh-so-obvious overtures. It had been a long time since a man had looked at me like that. Five years, to be exact.

But I was determined not to respond. Ben was great-looking and quite compelling, but I was a little bit *scared* of him. I certainly didn't know him very well. And most of what I had learned about him was stuff he had told me himself. All I could say for sure, from my own experience, was that he was rich and handsome and liked to smoke dope. For all I knew, he could be a white supremacist, or a child molester, or a drug dealer. He could even be Jane's *murderer*, for God's sake! I would *not*, under any circumstances, allow myself to become attracted to him.

But in the past few days my body had developed a control center of its own. Ben looked at me and a secret thrill started bubbling at the back of my brain, filling me with warmth as it oozed down to the base of my spine. I was thoroughly ashamed of myself.

Squirming with embarrassment, I gave Ben a weak smile and quickly changed the subject. "How long have you been divorced?" I asked him. The last time I mentioned the word divorce, he had gotten upset and introspective. I hoped it would have that effect again.

No such luck. Instead of retreating from my inquiry, Ben embraced it as a sign that I was eager to know more about his personal life. "Kate and I legally called it quits last year," he told me, "but the marriage was over long before then. She hated me for ruining her career, and I hated her for ruining my life. She was bored and bitchy and lousy in bed. And she couldn't even have any kids to relieve the boredom. We were married seventeen years, but it was a bust from the beginning."

"That's too bad," I said.

"Water under the bridge," he replied.

"Why did you leave Aspen and come back East?" I asked. Time for a new line of questioning.

"I just got sick of it. Sick of the whole divorce business—my clients' as well as my own. Sick of making money from other people's misery. Tired of expensive restaurants, ski slope wardrobes, luxury cars, and greedy young women." The marijuana had made him unusually talkative. "I couldn't hack it anymore," he went on. "Decided to chuck the whole mess and come back home, see if I still had any roots planted around here."

"And do you?"

"Nope. Don't belong here, either. I knew that after I was home for a week. Started looking around for work overseas. I'd like to live in London, I think. I haven't found anything yet, but I will soon. My father had a lot of friends in Europe." He brushed his fingers over his mustache and then rubbed his face and weary eyes with both hands.

"You must be exhausted," I said. "It's been a hard day."

"Yeah, right."

I saw the opening and leapt into it. "Well, I'd better be going home now," I declared, standing up and hoisting my purse over my shoulder. The filched Filofax seemed to weigh as much as an unabridged dictionary. "It was nice to see you again, Ben," I added. "I just wish it could have been under better circumstances." Sometimes clichés did have their uses.

"Well, let's make sure the next time *is* under better circumstances," he said, grinning. He rose to his feet, slipped his arm around my waist and began leading me across the veranda toward my car. "How about tomorrow night? Dinner at the Garden City Hotel. You can't beat *those* circumstances."

"I thought you were tired of expensive restaurants."

"I'll make an exception, just for you. Besides, this restaurant has the best Beef Wellington I've ever tasted in my life. And homemade ice cream with hot fudge sauce."

At this, a spurt of saliva flowed under my tongue. And more questions about Jane took shape in my mind. I told Ben I'd meet him in the hotel lounge at seven o'clock.

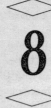

8

The Long Island Expressway is like life—straight here and curvy there, sometimes smooth and other times bumpy, often too fast but usually too slow, and always under construction. Driving home from the Masterson estate, I had to squeeze into single-lane traffic past two major work zones. I filled the time by mulling over the events of the day, and putting the new facts I had assembled into order.

I was amazed at how easy this detective work was turning out to be. All you had to do was get people to talk. And all you had to do to get people to talk was ask them questions about themselves. They'll keep talking as long as you keep listening. And I was a good listener. Always had been. At least that's what Sam used to tell me. "You've always got your ears turned on," he would say.

I was surprised but relieved that my discovery of Jane's body had never become a subject of that afternoon's conversation. Bette Masterson obviously had no idea who I was and Ben had been kind—or cunning—

enough not to mention my role in the ghastly chain of events surrounding Jane's death.

None of the people I met at the Masterson house that day had discerned my real motives for being there. I felt certain of that. No one had the slightest inkling I had come for any reason other than to pay my respects to the family. No one except, perhaps, the old woman named Daisy, who might have been shrieking, "You can't judge a book by its cover!" *about* me instead of *to* me.

But overall, I thought the first day of my own private murder investigation had gone very well. I had picked up a lot of pertinent information about the Masterson family—Ben and Jane in particular—and I was in an excellent position to get more. Dinner with Ben was sure to offer a good harvest, and I felt comfortable enough with Bette to visit her again soon. Maybe I'd get a chance to talk to Daisy, too. Or the Stanwycks, since they lived nearby.

I wasn't so afraid of being found out, or worried about what to say to people anymore. One of the most useful things I learned that day was that most people are so wrapped up in their own lives and intrigues they don't spend much time wondering about the lives and intrigues of others. As I looked back over the hours just passed, I realized that except for asking my name, not one person had made a single inquiry about *me* all afternoon.

It was only four o'clock—nowhere near dinnertime—but I made myself a tunafish sandwich and a bowl of vegetable soup as soon as I got home. While I was eating, my three cats, Groucho, Lucy, and Katy Kat—named after Groucho Marx, Lucille Ball, and nobody in particular—sat like watchdogs in the middle of the kitchen floor following every bite and spoonful with swiveling heads and half-closed yellow eyes. I knew their little stomachs had gotten excited the minute they heard the electric can opener, so after I emptied my bowl, I filled theirs with Happy Cat.

Then I walked—make that *limped*—into the bedroom to change my clothes. My aching, swollen feet felt like overstuffed duffel bags. I wondered how women who wear high heels to work every day keep from committing suicide every night.

As I was getting out of my dress and into my jeans and T-shirt, the phone rang. It was Philly.

"You're home early," I said to her.

"You got that right!" she exclaimed. "That detective friend of yours, Sergeant Frecklehead, came to the nursin' home this afternoon and sprang my ass outta there. Showed my supervisor his badge and said he was conductin' a murder investigation. Said I wasn't a suspect, but I would be tied up in questionin' for the rest of the day. Hon*eeey*! I wish you could've seen her eyes! They got as big as pizza pies. I'm talkin' *large*."

I laughed. "You'll be a celebrity at work tomorrow."

"I don't sign no autographs," she said, pretending annoyance.

I laughed again. "So what happened? Where did Eddie take you?"

"We went down to the parkin' lot and sat in his car. It didn't take long. And when we were finished I just jumped in my own car and came on home. Hope my nosy supervisor wasn't lookin' out the window."

"What questions did he ask?"

"Oh, just about what happened that night. What time we found the body. What we did when we found it. Stuff like that. He was real interested in why we were in the library together. Kept askin' me over and over why we met each other there and what we were doin'."

My stomach sank all the way down to my swollen feet. That was the *one* question Eddie had never asked *me*, and I knew Philly probably hadn't told him the truth. Like many LVA students, she hated to admit her reading problems to *anybody*. Only her sisters, Woodrow, and I knew that she had ever been illiterate. "What did you tell him?" I asked anxiously.

"I said we just liked to sit there and read encyclopedias together."

Philly and I had studied the word *encyclopedia* at one of our recent lessons, and once Philly learned to read and spell a word—especially, as she would say, a "big fat show-off word"—she liked to use it at every opportunity.

"Oh God, Philly! I wish you had told him the truth. He's never going to believe what you said. The idea that two grown women would meet in the library every week just to read encyclopedias together is preposterous!"

"Posterous? What's that posterous?"

"*Pre*posterous. P-r-e-p-o-s-t-e-r-o-u-s," I spelled out. "It means absurd, impossible to believe."

"Oh," she muttered.

"Never mind," I said quickly. I hated myself for embarrassing her. And I hated to poke holes in the fragile self-confidence I had worked so hard to build up. "It doesn't matter. I'm sure they don't still think I had anything to do with the murder. They've had four days to work on the case. They must have come up with some new leads by now."

"I sure do hope so, Annie," she said in a small, apologetic voice. "I'd let the cops pull out all my fingernails 'fore I'd say anything to hurt you."

Considering the unabashed pride Philly took in her long, manicured nails, that was saying a lot. "Don't you worry about a thing, chile," I teased, dredging up my long-lost Southern accent for her amusement. "And keep yo pretty fingernails in yo fingers where they belong. Ain't nobody gonna be hurtin' me!"

She giggled. "Hope dem words don't turn out to be yo famous *last* words," she said, exaggerating her own South Carolina drawl.

Self-confidence crisis over, I dropped my Southern accent and told Philly all about the funeral, and about my brave clue-hunting expedition to the Masterson estate afterward. I told her everything I'd learned about Jane and Ben and the other people I'd had a chance to observe. I thought she'd be proud of me for overcoming my scaredy-cat tendencies. I thought she'd be excited about what I found out. Instead, she pushed me into a slight self-confidence crisis of my own.

"Are you crazy, girl?" she cried. "You lookin' to get your head shot off, or somethin'? Whoever killed that poor kid has a *gun*, sugar, and from the looks of that great big hole in that little lady's body, he's not afraid to use it! You just *beggin'* for trouble, and you gonna get yourself in a whole mess of it. You better leave the detective work up to your frecklepuss boyfriend. At least *he* has his *own* gun!"

"But you don't understand! I wasn't in any danger at all. Everybody thought I was there just for the funeral. Nobody knows what I was doing."

"*Yet*, girlfriend. Nobody knows *yet*."

"Well, I appreciate your concern for me, Philly, but I think you're overreacting. If you'd been there you'd know there's nothing to worry about. Besides, I plan to be *very* careful. So let's just forget about it for now, okay?" I wanted to get off the subject before I freaked out and lost my nerve.

"Meanwhile," I added, "what are you going to do with this whole extra hour you've got on your hands? I'm sure you don't want to waste it talking to me."

"Oh, I'm just gonna lay down and take a nap. I'm as worn-out as a pair of old shoes. And I'm on hall watch tonight so I'll be up late."

Woodrow and Philly lived in a nice apartment in a not-so-nice Queens neighborhood. In an effort to keep their building safe at night, all the able-bodied tenants took turns policing the halls. Philly was on watch, stationed in a chair right by the stairwell and the elevators, from seven to ten every Monday night. And she was worried about me! For three hours a week, every week, she put herself at risk to guard her neighbors' safety. And at any moment during those three hours she could find herself nose to nose with a gun.

"Well, you'd better hang up and hit the sack, kiddo," I said. "You don't want to doze off out there in the hall tonight."

"That would never happen," she insisted. "I won't be sleepin', I'll be *readin'*."

After Philly and I hung up, I flopped down on my back on the bed and, stretching my left leg out to its full extension, turned on the TV with my toe. *Live at Five*, a news show on channel four—I always thought they should call it *Live at Five on Four*—was on.

Crime was up. Employment was down. The national debt was staying the same. Hemlines and welfare lines were getting longer, while water supplies and the president's temper were getting shorter. The San Andreas fault, the Mount St. Helen volcano, and Saddam Hussein were all acting up again.

I was about to close my eyes for a catnap when Jane's face appeared on the screen and snapped me back to attention. "Nassau County police are still looking for leads in the shooting death of 26-year-old Jane Camille Masterson, whose naked body was found in the trunk of a car parked in the Hempstead Library lot last Thursday night," the newscaster reported. "Anyone with any information relating to the case is asked to call the Homicide Department at Nassau County Police Headquarters. All calls will be kept confidential."

I was wide awake then, and figured I probably would be for the rest of the night. If the police were putting out TV appeals like this, that meant they probably weren't any closer to catching the killer than they were last Friday when I was questioned by Lieutenant O'Donnell. What the hell was going on? I suddenly wondered why Eddie hadn't been at the funeral today, and why the cops hadn't confiscated Jane's Filofax. Why was it taking them so long to get on the right track in this case?

More questions I couldn't answer. I jumped up, grabbed my purse off the dresser and plopped it down on the bed next to me. Then I took out the stolen Filofax and began flipping through the pages, one at a time.

There wasn't a single entry in the diary section and all the pages provided for notes and memos were blank. The month-at-a-glance calendar was also devoid of markings. A few random equations—simple additions and subtractions—appeared in the financial records section and the numerous pages of the daily appointment calendar contained only those few notations I had seen earlier, when I first found the book in Jane's bedroom. The address and telephone directory offered just two listings: Niles, 883-0492; and Rebirth, 208 E. 67th St., (212) 422-9864.

I closed the book in dismay. No wonder the police hadn't bothered taking the darn thing back to Headquarters—there wasn't anything in it! I had become a common thief and risked having a major heart attack for nothing. Well, not for *nothing* exactly. At least now I had Niles Stanwyck's phone number, which would save me looking it up. And now I also knew, or so it seemed, that Rebirth was the *name* of something—some kind of practice or business in the city—not just a cutesy license plate.

Big deal. Those two phone numbers certainly weren't worth the tampering with evidence charge that could, I realized with a spasm of panic, be leveled against me in a court of law. I wondered if I should try to sneak back into Jane's room and return the book to her desk drawer. *Or maybe*, I thought hysterically, *I should destroy it altogether!* I saw myself dressed all in black and creeping out into the backyard after midnight to set the Filofax on fire. Then I imagined taking a little trip over to Staten Island and throwing the damn thing off the Verrazano Bridge.

Finally, I put the book on a shelf in my closet, behind a stack of old sweatshirts. Then I stretched out on the bed again and took several deep breaths, trying to forget it was there. With my eyes squeezed shut, my hands balled into fists and my body as relaxed as a surfboard, I tried to put several other troubling thoughts out of my mind as well: that Philly had lied to Eddie about what we were doing in the library; that the police probably still thought I had something to do with Jane's death; that the real murderer was still on the loose, with his gun and his good name intact.

When the doorbell rang an hour later, I was working myself up into an all-out anxiety attack. I tried to ignore the bell, but it rang again and again. I didn't want to open the door. The way my luck was going, there had to be something bad on the other side. For one insane moment I thought it must be the killer, coming after *me*.

It was Eddie. And he looked terrible. His face was pale—except for the freckled parts. His hair was damp and disheveled, and his shoulders drooped as if they'd been deflated. Even his clothes looked limp.

"What happened to you?" I asked, opening the door wide enough for him to enter. "You look like Dick Tracy after a tough night in a trash masher."

"I haven't slept much lately," he said, stepping inside and sweeping his glassy eyes around the living room.

"Well, what can I do for you? Fix you a cup of coffee? Loan you a pillow?"

"Coffee sounds good."

"Come with me," I said, leading the way into the kitchen and directing him to a chair at the table. "Are you hungry?" I asked as I put some water up to boil. "I've got some leftover tuna salad. I could make you a sandwich." It's really revolting how *some* women will knock themselves silly trying to prove their happy little homemaker skills to men they find attractive.

"A sandwich would be great," he said. "I've got at least two hours of paperwork back at the office before I go home for dinner." He propped one elbow on the table, rested his chin in his hand and watched me measure instant coffee into my Mickey and Minnie Mouse mugs.

"I didn't see you at the funeral this morning," I said.

"I couldn't make it. I had to meet Claudine and the kids at the airport. They landed at Kennedy a little before eleven."

"Oh." I resisted the urge to scowl.

"Detective Fred Spockett—better known as Spock—went in my place. He said he saw you there."

"Oh?"

"He went to the funeral, the graveside service, and back to the house afterward. Said you were there too."

"Yeah," I admitted. I cut Eddie's sandwich in half and almost sliced my finger in the process. Some detective *I* was turning out to be. I couldn't even spot another detective snooping around in the same vicinity, watching *me*. I wondered if Spock had followed me upstairs and seen me go into Jane's room.

"What does Detective Spockett look like?" I asked, trying to sound cool, calm, and casual. "I didn't notice him there. Does he have pointy ears?"

"Medium height and weight, about fifty, gray hair, normal ears. Probably wearing a dark suit and tie."

No wonder I didn't notice him. He looked like every other man at the funeral. Every one except Ben. I put Eddie's sandwich plate down on the table in front of him and poured boiling water into our coffee mugs. "Why didn't he talk to me? Shouldn't he have introduced himself or something?" I asked.

"Well, to be perfectly honest with you," Eddie said, gulping down a mouthful of tunafish, "he was there to keep an eye on *you* as much as anybody else. Wouldn't make sense for him to tell you who he was."

I tried to keep myself under control, but I couldn't.

"God!" I cried. "I can't believe I'm still a suspect in this case!" Then I really lost it. "If you guys would stop wasting so much time watching *me*," I shouted, "maybe you'd be able to figure out who the *real* killer is!"

"Take it easy, Annie. You shouldn't get so upset. We're just going by the book here. It's routine procedure."

"Yeah, well, your routine procedure really sucks!" I said, shocking myself with my own vulgarity. "And, even worse, it's incredibly stupid. I mean, shouldn't you and your detective buddies be focusing your brilliant investigative powers on the *men* in Jane's life? The girl was *raped*, for God's sake! How the hell could *I* have done *that*?"

Eddie stopped eating and looked at me through suddenly narrow eyes. And when he spoke his tone was angry. "How did you know she was raped? That information was never released to *anybody*. Not even the family."

I couldn't breathe. I couldn't even see straight. Everything looked fuzzy and kind of wiggly. Why did I have to be born with a tongue? Couldn't that part have been left out? Why was I ever born at all? I took a sip of my coffee and tried to think. Not that I had anything worthwhile to think *with*.

"I didn't know she was raped," I said finally. "I just assumed she was since she was naked."

I looked at Eddie's face to see if he believed me, but I couldn't tell if he bought my explanation or not. He looked as if he didn't know *what* to believe. I considered telling him about the conversation I'd overheard while sitting in O'Donnell's office, but decided against it. I wasn't ready to relinquish the little edge of knowledge and power I had barely managed to gain.

"So I was right, huh? She *was* raped." I gave Eddie a sly smile, hoping to promote the impression that I had tricked him into revealing the rape to me. My ruse seemed to work.

"Yes," he admitted, looking confused.

"So, then, since she was raped by a man, and I am obviously *not* a man, would you mind telling me why *I'm* still under suspicion?"

"She could have been raped and murdered by two different people," Eddie said simply. "Or the rapist/murderer could have had an accomplice, someone to help him dispose of the body."

I was feeling pretty sick by then. And very, very dumb. Why had none of these possibilities occurred to me before? "So," I stumbled on, "you think I helped the murderer get rid of the body by loading it into my car trunk and driving it to the Hempstead Library?"

"As I told you before," Eddie said, "*I* don't think you had anything to do with it. But I'm not the only homicide detective working on this case. Lieutenant O'Donnell has a few hunches of his own. And now Spock's getting into the act, bringing new information to the table."

"New information? What new information?"

"I shouldn't be telling you this," Eddie said, "but Spock's gotten it into his head that you and Ben Masterson are pretty thick. Thick as thieves, he thinks. He said the two of you sat outside on the porch together for most of the afternoon. Looked like you were all wrapped up in a private conversation, and maybe in each other, too." Eddie was watching me intently, waiting for my reaction.

I just sat there and stared at my coffee mug. I was starting to feel numb; and afraid to say anything more. Afraid that if I opened my mouth one of my feet would jump back in there and start kicking the hell out of whatever credibility I had left. Finally I mumbled something about Ben and I renewing our old acquaintance and talking about old times. "I was just being polite," I explained.

Amazingly, this seemed to satisfy him. "I figured it was something like that," he said. He downed the rest of his coffee and rose to his feet. "Better get a move on. As it is, I won't get home till after nine. Claudine and the kids will be upset, their first night back and all."

"Can't you go straight home and leave the paperwork for the morning?"

"No. Gotta get everything down while it's fresh in my mind." I followed him to the front door. "Thanks for the sandwich," he said. As tired and conflicted as he was, Eddie still radiated an aura of strength and dependability. He was, I thought, the kind of man who would always take care of business.

I opened the door for him and he stepped out on the porch. "Please keep me posted on any new developments, okay?" I asked. "Since I'm still under suspicion, I think I have a right to know what's going on."

"Well, that's not really true, Annie," he said. "Sometimes the success of an investigation will hinge on its total secrecy."

"Isn't it a law that a suspect has to be kept apprised of what he or she is being suspected of?" I didn't know what I was saying, but I thought it sounded good.

"Gee, I never heard of a law like that," he said, breaking out in a great big, goofy grin. "Guess I'd better go to the library and look it up in the *encyclopedia*." A devilish flash of merriment shot out of his tired eyes. Then he turned his fabulous self around and headed down the front walk to his car.

9

Some call it sleep, but I call it a semiconscious state of flopping around in bed all night, dozing a little, dreaming a little and worrying a lot.

I had two dreams that night. In the first one Eddie and I were getting married, in the same church where Jane's funeral had been held. Eddie was wearing a tuxedo, but I was wearing a black bikini. My late husband was performing the ceremony. "Do you take this man?" Sam asked me, but before I could answer, he grabbed me by the arm and pushed me down behind the pulpit. Then a shot rang out from the back of the church, and Eddie fell down dead at the altar, with a clean, bloodless hole through his neck the size of a quarter.

The second dream started with a sex scene—Ben and I making out in the backseat of a black limo. The TV was on, filling the passenger area with wavy light and the musical theme from *Star Trek*. Ben had unbuttoned my blouse and he was covering my neck and shoulders with soft, hot kisses. But all of a sudden he got crazy. He started pushing me down on the seat and trying to rip off my black lace bra. Just then Eddie yanked open the car door, pulled Ben off of me, and put us both under arrest. We were marched off to jail, through a field of blue flowers, with our hands cuffed behind our backs.

Between dreams, and between the recurrent bouts of anguish over the murder and everything connected with it, I worried about every other little detail of my life, from what I was going to have for breakfast in the morning, to whether or not my computer was infected with a virus. At eight o'clock, when I wrenched my piti-ful body out of the bed, I felt as anxious and jittery as if I'd spent the night in a Roach Motel.

I took a shower, had coffee, ate a banana, took two aspirin, and went to the gym. After a half-hour on the treadmill and twenty minutes on the upper body machines, I went home and took another shower. By then I was starting to feel normal again. Well, not exactly *normal*, but like my old self at least. My old, nor-mally anxious self.

I had a salad for lunch and then sat down at the com-puter to finish up an assignment for *Redbook*, a short filler called "How to Look Like a Million Bucks on a Penny Pincher's Budget"—as if *I* knew anything about that! (The million bucks part, I mean. When it came to pennies, I could outpinch Scrooge McDuck.) I had been working for about an hour when the phone rang. Groaning out loud, I jumped up and went dashing around the house looking for the portable phone. It was in the living room on the piano.

"I'm glad I caught you at home," Ben said. "I'm in the car on the way into the city to see a couple of people about jobs, and I wanted to make sure that we're still on for tonight."

"We're on," I said, pacing around the coffee table and peering through the picture window at the sky. The day was turning dark and cloudy. So was my mood. The thought of meeting Ben for dinner was making me nervous again.

"Great," he said. "Seven o'clock in the hotel lounge, right?"

"Right."

"Good. My last appointment is at four. It should only take an hour or so. I'll head straight for the hotel as soon as it's over."

"Fine. I'll see you then."

Turning off the phone, I carried it with me back to my office to keep near the computer while I was working. But before I even sat down at my desk again, I had completely changed my plans for the afternoon. My freelance article could wait. It didn't have a specific deadline. What *couldn't* wait was my next visit to the Masterson estate. Ben was going to be gone for the whole afternoon, and I didn't want to waste such a perfect opportunity to talk to Bette, and hopefully Daisy, without his interference.

After shutting down the Mac, I darted into the bathroom, brushed my hair and slathered on some makeup. Getting dressed as quickly as I could in a black knit pantsuit and a yellow tube top, I put on some gold hoop earrings and those damn high heels again. I figured I'd better dress up enough for dinner in case I couldn't make it home in time to change.

Forty-five minutes later I was pulling into the long, winding cobblestone drive to the Masterson house. Thick gray clouds were still darkening the sky, making the deep green lawns and trees look even deeper and greener. I parked the car in front this time and walked quickly up the pachysandra-lined path to the main entrance. Sucking in a chestful of air, I rang the doorbell.

After a few moments a maid answered. It was the same quick-thinking woman who had, after Daisy's shocking outburst the day before, saved the old girl—and the open-mouthed guests—from further embarrassment with the promise of a cherry soda. I could tell she recognized me.

"I'm here to see Mrs. Masterson," I told her. "My name is Annie March. Bette isn't expecting me, but I was in the neighborhood and I thought she might like to have some company for a little while."

"That's nice," she said, smiling. "Come inside and I'll tell her you're here. You can have a seat if you like." She pointed to an ornate wooden chair sitting next to an equally ornate table in the hall. "I hope you'll understand if she's indisposed or too tired to receive you."

"Of course," I said, sitting down.

While the maid was gone I tried to think of a painless way to get Bette to talk about Jane. But painless would be impossible, I soon realized. I remembered all too well how I'd felt after Sam's death, and I knew Bette would plunge into agony with every mention of her dead daughter's name. Shortly the maid reappeared.

"Mrs. Masterson will be glad to see you," she announced. "You can visit with her in her bedroom. If you'll just follow me . . ." She led me across the hall and up the curving blue-carpeted staircase. I didn't tell her that I already knew the way.

Bette was sitting in a plump armchair with a plaid wool blanket over her lap. She wore brown velvet slippers on her tiny feet, which peeked out from under the blanket like twin Chihuahuas. On top of the table next to her chair were two paperback romances, a glass of water, and about eighty bottles of pills.

"It's lovely to see you again, dear," she said, slowly lifting her thin white arm and quivering hand in greeting. "Come. Sit down here, next to me." She motioned me to a small settee placed next to her chair, facing the cold fireplace. "Linda," she said to the maid, "would you bring us some tea please? There's such a chill in the air today."

"Yes, Mrs. Masterson," Linda replied, exiting the room.

"I think I'll go downstairs and have a cup of tea myself," said a deep female voice behind me. I turned to see a large-boned woman in a white uniform emerging from the shadows near the large four-poster bed. Her hair was pinned up in a bun and her face was the shape of a shoe box.

"Of course, Dora," Bette said. "Take as long as you like. You deserve a break."

Bette watched her leave the bedroom as a baby might watch her mother leave the nursery. "Dora's the best day nurse I've ever had," she said to me. "She's leaving next month for a job in California, and I don't know what I'm going to do without her. It's so hard to find good help these days," she sighed, voicing the timeless lament of the wealthy. "Nobody even speaks English anymore."

"I know," I said, as if the search for proper servants had also been *my* cross to bear. The only kind of help I'd ever hired had been a housepainter, and a neighborhood kid to cut the grass.

"Daisy will miss Dora, too," Bette added. "She's become so attached to her she follows her around like a little puppy. I haven't told Daisy that Dora's going away yet. I can't bear to upset her. Since the accident she's had so little control over her emotions."

"You mentioned an accident to me yesterday," I said, glad for the chance to reopen the subject. "What kind of accident was it?"

"You mean you don't know? I thought everybody with any connection to our family knew all about it by now."

"Well, Ben and I sort of lost touch over the years," I said, hoping that would explain my ignorance and encourage Bette to elaborate.

It did. Bette rested her head against the back of her chair, stared intently into the middle of the room and began speaking in a soft, hypnotic voice. "It happened over ten years ago," she said. "In the summer. Daisy and her husband, Schuyler, were both fifty-four at the time. They had been married for thirty-five years, and you never saw a happier couple in your life. They were so much in love it made your heart feel good just to look at them.

"They were best friends, too. Had been ever since Sky moved into the house next door, just before Daisy's tenth birthday. They were always together and they never dated anybody else all through high school. They got married right after graduation. Daisy had some sort of blockage in her fallopian tubes, so they never had any children, but that never bothered them one bit. All Daisy and Sky ever needed was each other.

"Sky owned his own hardware business," Bette went on, "and Daisy helped him out at the store, writing correspondence, doing the books and such. And whenever they could get a few days off they'd take an automobile trip together. They just loved to get in the car and go!

They'd drive up to the Catskills, or out to the South Fork, or down to Amish country. They drove all the way out to the Grand Canyon once. If they weren't in the store, or at home in their house in Scarsdale, they were in their old green Lincoln convertible driving all over creation and back.

"It was on one of their little trips—to Connecticut, I think it was—that the accident occurred." Bette screwed the wrinkles of her soft white face into a hard black scowl. "They were driving down the highway with the top down when a sudden thunderstorm broke out and pounded the area with torrential rains. Sky lost control of the car, skidding partially *under* an enormous tractor trailer truck to his left. The upper part of the driver's side of the car was demolished and poor Schuyler was decapitated."

"Oh my God!" I cried. I could barely imagine such a scene. Somewhere in the distance a burglar alarm went off and a dog started howling.

"My sister wasn't hurt at all," Bette continued, still staring into the middle of the room and speaking in a near whisper. "There wasn't a scratch on her. Not even a bruise. But, for Daisy, that just made everything worse. I can't help thinking that she'd be better off if she'd lost an arm or a leg. Maybe then she wouldn't have had to lose her mind."

"Lose her mind?"

"When help arrived and they pulled Daisy out of the car, she was singing and talking and giggling to herself like a young girl. The doctors later decided that she had regressed to the age of nine—the age she was before she ever knew Schuyler.

"And she's been like that ever since?"

"Yes. After months and months of analysis, Daisy's

doctors came to the conclusion that, in order to block out the unbearable memory of Sky's horrible death, Daisy had to forget that she'd ever known him at all. So she simply became nine years old again and erased all traces of Schuyler from her mind. Unfortunately, she had to erase the rest of her memory as well."

"That's awful," I said. "I'm so sorry."

"Yes . . . well . . . the hard part for me is that she doesn't realize I'm her sister. Daisy was thirteen when I was born, and now she doesn't remember me, or our past life together, at all."

"Here we are!" Linda chirped, interrupting our sad conversation. She carried a large silver tray into the room and placed it on the coffee table in front of the settee. The tray held a china teapot, matching cups and saucers, and a platter of sugar cookies with pink frosting. "I've brought you some tea, some cookies, and some company," she said, looking over her shoulder at the short chubby white-haired figure standing in the doorway.

"Can I come in?" Daisy called out.

"Of course, dear," Bette answered. "We're about to have some tea. Would you like some?"

"No, thank you, ma'am," Daisy politely replied, bouncing into the room and plopping down on a footstool near the coffee table. She was wearing a baby-blue sweatshirt, baggy jeans, and high-top sneakers with glitter glued all over them. "I'll just have a cookie," she said, leaning over the edge of the table and snatching the top one off the pile. She looked over at me with a big grin, licked off all the pink icing, and then ate the cookie.

"This is Mrs. March," Bette said to her, nodding in my direction. "She was here yesterday. Do you remember her?"

"Sure I do. She's the deaf one."

"What?" Bette said.

"When Daisy spoke to me yesterday I was having a little trouble with my hearing," I quickly explained. "But I'm all better now."

"Oh . . . hmmm . . . that's nice," Bette murmured.

"You're pretty," Daisy said, staring at me with squinty eyes. "You look just like Snow White. I love that movie! I've seen it twice. Remember when Snow White was lost in the forest and all the animals came out and sat in her lap? That was my favorite part."

"Mine too!" I said, really meaning it. I had always loved the birds and bunnies in that scene.

"You know what else I like?" Daisy said, grabbing another cookie and licking off the frosting. "I like Jane's flowers. She made the most beautiful flowers in the world."

"She did?" I asked, hoping to keep her talking about Jane.

"Oh yes!" Daisy exclaimed. Her girlish black eyes sparkled in her old woman's face. "And she made all different kinds, too. I don't remember all the names she told me. I just remember sweetpeas and snapdragons 'cause their names are so cute. You wanna come outside with me? I'll show you where the best ones are growing. And I'll take you out to the greenhouse where all the pots and the seeds and the little baby plants are."

"I'd love to," I said, looking over at Bette for approval. She nodded sadly. She was exhausted, I realized, and anxious for us to leave. And she was hoping, no doubt, that the thought of Jane and her beautiful flowers would go away with us.

"Okay, let's go!" Daisy commanded, jumping to her sneakered feet and dancing an impatient little jig on the floor in front of the fireplace. At sixty-six, she had more energy than most of the women in my aerobics class, including me.

I stood up, said good-bye to Bette and told her I would visit again soon. Then I followed Daisy out of the room. Behind us, I could hear Bette pouring herself a cup of tea. Her hand shook so violently the lid of the teapot rattled like tiny china bones.

"The best flowers are out by the greenhouse," Daisy said as we left the house through the back door and headed down the path to the parking area. "There's blue ones and lavender ones and a lot of yellow ones. Jane let *me* help plant all the blubs!"

"Blubs?" I wondered.

"Yeah! You know! Those hard round brown things? You dig a hole and you put in some fertilizer. Then you stick the blub in and cover it up with dirt. It's easy!"

"Oh, *now* I know what you mean," I said. "But I think they're called *bulbs,* not blubs."

"Well, whatever you call 'em, they're blooming great!" she whooped, unaware of her amusing play on words. "Come on! They're out by the gardener's room and the tool shed." She struck out, half skipping and half walking, across the yard toward the greenhouse. I followed along as quickly as I could, my high heels poking little holes in the perfect lawn.

"See!" she cried when we reached the far side of the white wood and glass outbuilding. "Aren't they beautiful?"

And indeed they were. Rows and rows of irises, from the deepest blue imaginable to the lightest shade of lilac, lined the far side of the recessed, brick-walled garden, and a dazzling sea of yellow daffodils filled the rest of the arena. Thick patches of dark green ivy climbed up and over the mossy brick borders.

"This was one of Jane's favorite gardens," Daisy said, suddenly turning sad. "She loved those big blue flowers best of all. She liked to cut them and bring them into the house. And she always brought some for my room."

"Were you and Jane good friends?" I asked her.

"Yes, ma'am!" she exclaimed. "I loved her more than anybody else in the world. I don't know why she had to die. I can't believe I'm never going to see her again."

"Do you remember what you were doing the night she died?"

"I was drawing pictures and watching TV."

"Where was Jane?"

"I don't know. In her room, I guess."

"Did you see or hear anything funny that night? Did you see any strange people or hear any screaming or shooting?"

"You mean on TV?"

"No, I mean for real."

"No!" she cried. "Why would I hear any screaming or shooting? That's just crazy!"

"Do you know how Jane died?"

"Sure I do. She went to sleep and never woke up."

"Oh, I see. But do you know how or why she went to sleep?"

"She was just tired, I guess." Daisy's eyes welled up with tears and her chin started quivering. "But I don't see *why* she had to be so tired! She went to bed early every night and she could sleep as late as she wanted to. It was all those stupid damn operations, I bet!" she said, suddenly turning angry. "Every time she'd get an operation she'd come home all bandaged up and tired and stay in bed for days." Daisy's face got red and she started kicking at the ground so hard her sneakers sprinkled silver glitter on the grass.

Not wanting to send the old woman into a fit, I patted her back and shoulders and hastily changed the subject. "Can we go inside the greenhouse now?" I asked. "I'd like to see the little baby plants you mentioned."

"Okay," she said, relaxing under my touch and leaning against my side. To my surprise, she put her arms around me and squeezed hard. "You're nice," she said, looking up at me with such a loving expression it almost broke my heart.

Daisy took me by the hand and led me away from the bulb garden. As we walked around the large tool shed and neared the door to the main greenhouse, we passed the wide-open windows of the gardener's quarters—a small room with a wooden floor, a desk, a chair, a little refrigerator, a portable TV, and an army-blanketed cot in the corner. The TV was turned on and tuned in to *Live at Five*. I could tell by the familiar voices of the newscasters. The door was open and a dark-haired young man with an olive complexion and a thick black mustache stuck his head out as we walked by. He had a dirty white handkerchief tied around his neck.

"Hi, Juan!" Daisy called out to him, frantically waving her free hand. Juan waved back, but didn't answer.

"That's the groundskeeper," Daisy told me under her breath as we walked on. "He works here every day and sometimes he has other people come in to help him with the mowing and big cleanups. He could live here if he wanted to, but he lives somewhere else with his wife and children. He's got about six little kids. But I don't think he likes it at home 'cause lots of nights he stays here late, even when he doesn't have to. I came out and spent the evening with him a couple of times. It was fun. We watched TV and ate corn chips and drank big cans of Dr. Pepper."

Still holding my hand, Daisy pulled me through the entrance to the greenhouse. The enormous old building was wonderfully maintained. The waist-high walls and wooden window frames looked newly painted and all of the glass panes, even those in the vaulted roof, were crystal clean. Long redwood tray tables laden with clay-potted plants sat in wall-to-wall rows, with narrow aisles and wooden boardwalks in between. The boardwalks seemed to have been custom-made, with half-inch spaces between two-inch wood strips and a deep layer of brownish-red pebbles underneath. I could hardly walk there in my pumps.

"Isn't it neat in here?" Daisy asked. "I love the damp, warmy feeling and the way the air smells like dirt and perfume all mixed up together. Come this way!" she cried, bounding down the redwood runner to the right. "The best stuff is down here!"

Struggling to keep my heels from getting stuck between the slats, I followed Daisy to the far end of the greenhouse. The tables on each side of the aisle were filled to capacity with plants and flowers of all sizes, shapes, and colors, and many different species of ferns dangled in plastic planters from sturdy, strategically placed wooden beams. There was a closed door at the end of that particular walkway which led, I decided, to Juan's domain.

"Looky here!" Daisy said, picking up a small pot of sparkle ivy and holding it out to me. "Isn't it neat the way the leaves look like stars? And I like this one a lot, too," she said, stretching her squat body up on tiptoes and touching the ends of a hanging asparagus fern. "It's so light and fuzzy. If angels had green hair, I think it'd look just like this."

Daisy led me around the greenhouse for a while, pointing out her favorite plants and explaining her reasons for liking them. And the more time I spent in her childlike company, the more reasons I had for liking *her*.

"Can I ask you a question?" I said to Daisy as she walked me around to my car at the front of the house. "Remember yesterday when you came over to me and said, 'You can't judge a book by its cover'?"

"Yeah, sure."

"Did you mean anything special by that? Were you trying to tell me something?"

"Oh, I don't know," she said, taking hold of my hand again and playing with my thin gold pinkie ring. "It's just that I was standing there in the dining room after the funeral trying not to cry. I knew if I started, I wouldn't be able to stop, and I didn't want to look like a big baby. So, just to keep my mind busy, I started thinking about how different Jane was on the outside from the inside. I mean, after she had her operations and bleached her hair and all, she looked just like a model or a famous movie star on the outside. But on the inside she still felt like a lonely brown-haired fat girl with a big ugly nose. I know that's true 'cause she told me so."

Daisy looked up at the sky and her face became as dark as the thickening clouds overhead. "So I was standing there thinking about Jane," she went on, "and then I started looking around at all the dumb old phonies who went to her funeral and came back to the house acting so sad and upset. They all looked like they were gonna fall right over and die themselves! But I knew that most of them didn't even *know* Jane, or care about her *at all*. So I was starting to get real mad. And I was getting ready to yell at them and tell them all to go home and leave us alone.

"But then you walked in," she said with a smile. "And you looked *different* from everybody else. You looked like a *real* person, and I wanted to talk to you. So I just went over and told you what was on my mind. I would've stood and talked to you longer but I got thirsty and went to get a cherry soda."

"Oh," I said, suddenly feeling guilty about the less-than-honest role *I* had been playing. I looked into Daisy's sweet eyes and wondered how she would feel if she knew my real reasons for being there, talking with her, asking her questions and listening to her like a friend. I hoped she would understand, and I made a promise to myself to come back and see her often, after this whole mess was over.

Until that time, however, I still had some deceptive detective work to do. "What about Ben?" I asked her, raising my eyebrows in what I hoped was an innocent expression. "Do you think *his* book is different from *his* cover?"

"Oh sure! On the outside he acts like nothing ever bothers him—like he doesn't care *what* happens. And he talks like he doesn't give a fig about anything or anybody. But on the inside he's real scared, I think, and hiding from something." Daisy let go of my hand and began twisting a curl of white hair around her index finger. "You know what he reminds me of?" she said, snickering. "A boy who hurt his little sister on purpose and is hiding from his mother under the bed."

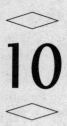

10

As soon as I pulled out of the Masterson driveway I started checking my rearview mirror, watching for Spock—which was pretty silly since I didn't know what Spock looked like. Still, I figured I'd better keep an eye out for a nondescript middle-aged man, with gray hair and normal ears, wearing a drab suit and driving a humdrum car. And if such a vision materialized behind me, I decided, I would take off like the Roadrunner and leave the old coyote in the dust. I certainly didn't want Spock following me to the hotel and finding out about my dinner date with Ben—much less spying on us!

After I had gone a half-mile down the road I noticed a dark blue Chevy with a gray-haired male driver pull into the line of traffic behind me. When I made a right turn onto Middle Neck Road, the blue Chevy did the same. The driver stayed on my tail, one or two cars back, all the way past the Sands Point Park and Preserve. I had no way of knowing if it was Spock or not, but to be on the safe side, I made a sharp right turn onto Radcliffe Avenue and stomped on the gas pedal.

I zoomed into familiar territory then—the Terrace section of Port Washington where I had lived during my high school years—and I knew my way around those twisting and unpredictable side streets as well as I knew the layout of my own kitchen. Whizzing down the hill like a bat out of hell, I peeled off onto Pepperday and tore past the small yellow ranch house my family had lived in. I hung a right at the corner, zipped up Avenue C for one block, and pulled another sharp right turn onto Glamford Avenue.

In the middle of the block, I screeched into an open parking spot at the curb. Then I turned off the ignition and scrunched down in my seat, gasping for air and shivering like a sparrow in shock. I had never driven so recklessly before. And I certainly had never tried to out-race a police detective before!

After a few moments of breathless stupefaction, I mustered the nerve to sit up straight and look out the window. The blue Chevy was nowhere in sight. I couldn't believe it! I had lost the sucker! My first car-chase scene, and *I* had been the winner!—assuming, of course, that Detective Spockett had actually been following me. My head reeled with the excitement and stupidity of it all. A middle-aged widow tear-assing around quiet suburban streets, risking life and limb—and the lives and limbs of all passing pedestrians—as if her freedom depended on it. And the sick part was, I realized, that maybe my freedom *did* depend on it.

With this sobering thought in mind, I decided to go visit my father for a little while instead of driving straight to the Garden City Hotel. I had some time to spare, I was in the right neighborhood, and I wanted to make double-sure that I wasn't being tailed. I pulled my little black Shadow away from the curb, drove up to the corner and took a left back onto Radcliffe. Then I slowly and carefully cruised the few blocks to the apartment complex where my father now lived, keeping watch in the rearview mirror all the way.

Daddy wasn't home. I rang his bell a few times, but got no response, so I let myself into his apartment with the key I keep in my purse at all times, just in case. I went to the bathroom—my wild ride had almost made me wet my pants—poured myself a Coke, and sat down at the table in the dining area.

Looking through the drawers of the bureau for a pencil and paper so I could leave my father a note, I spotted the little local phone directory. On a whim I picked it up and looked up Dr. Stanwyck. To my surprise, a complete listing was printed, giving his home number, office number, and Sands Point address.

When I found a pencil and a notepad, I wrote all the information down and stuffed the piece of paper into my purse. Then, after dashing off a quick note to my father, I detached the local map stapled inside the front cover of the phone book and jammed that into my purse as well. You never know when a good map will come in handy. Especially if you're searching for a murderer and don't know which way to turn.

The drive to Garden City was uneventful. No signs of Spock and, therefore, no whiplash detours. When I hit Old Country Road it started raining, and I cursed the loss of my big red umbrella—which was still sitting, I figured, on the back seat of my BMW, in the darkest and driest recesses of a locked and guarded Nassau County Police garage.

But I didn't need it, as it turned out. When I pulled up under the overhang of the main entrance to the hotel, a uniformed doorman wearing a dark green top hat and carrying an unnecessary umbrella came to usher me inside, and a slicker-clad valet whisked my car off to the parking lot. I passed through the heavy glass doors and into the lobby without a single raindrop splotching my shoulder. After a brief survey of the lobby's beige marble floors and enormous crystal and gold chandelier, I headed for the cocktail lounge—a darkened, carpeted, brass-railed platform of tables and chairs to the right.

As far as I could tell, Ben hadn't arrived yet. Almost every seat at the bar was taken and most of the tables were occupied by a coifed and bejeweled assortment of elderly millionaires and pampered preppie types. I stepped up into the lounge and sat down at a small round table, on a plush purple velvet banquette facing the hotel entrance. Within seconds a tall young waitress with very long red hair and a very short red skirt appeared at my side. I ordered a dry martini with five olives in it.

"Are you thirsty or hungry?" she asked, giggling.

"Both," I lied. I wasn't thirsty at all. I just wanted a light snack and a heavy sedative.

Before the waitress returned with my drink, I saw Ben push his way through the entrance doors into the hotel lobby. He breezed to the center of the beige marble floor, his black silk raincoat billowing behind him like Dracula's cape. I expected him to bear right and head for the lounge to look for me, but he turned to the left and went over to the registration desk instead.

Resting his elbows on top of the marble counter, he leaned over and said something to the pretty brunette behind the desk. She gave him a big sparkly smile and punched something into her computer. Then she nodded, said a few words, fluttered her eyelashes and gave him another big smile. He took out his wallet and handed her a credit card. She punched something else into her computer, went into the rear office, came out again and handed Ben his credit card plus a small white envelope. He put the card back into his wallet and shoved the envelope deep into the pocket of his raincoat. *Then* he headed for the bar.

I was sitting in the darkest, most remote corner of the cocktail lounge, so he didn't see me at first. He might not have seen me at all if the redheaded waitress in the short red skirt hadn't walked right by him on the way to deliver my drink. Captured by the spectacle of her bright red behind and following its progress across the floor to my table, his eyes eventually landed on me.

Ben cocked his head in surprise, sauntered over to my table and slid in next to me on the banquette. "You're early," he said, slipping his right arm around my shoulders. "I'll have a Jack Daniels and soda," he said to the waitress, giving her a wink and a slow once-over.

She smoldered in the heat of his attention. Even in the near-darkness I could see her pale white face flame to crimson. I felt a quick stab of jealousy followed by a tidal wave of self-disgust. Why were lascivious, controlling, insensitive guys like Ben always so irresistible to women? And why the hell was *I* susceptible to his cold-blooded, broad-shouldered charms? I'd always thought I was too smart and too sensible to find a thug like Ben appealing.

It probably had something to do with natural law, I reasoned (or rationalized, maybe). That whole survival of the fittest routine. Ben was strong, handsome, rich, and ruthless—obviously fit to survive. Women couldn't help being attracted to him. Nature had programmed them to respond. And, given enough time and enticement, most women would eventually consent to performing the baby-making act with him. It was natural selection. It was propagation of the species. It was the dumb, stupid, inescapable order of things.

"Been here long?" Ben asked, turning his dark brown eyes and attention to me as the waitress walked away.

"Just a few minutes."

"Good. I hate to keep a woman waiting."

I'll just bet you do, I said to myself.

"We're both gonna have to wait a while for dinner, though," he added, smiling his crooked smile and fingering his earring. He had changed from a gold stud to a small gold hoop. "The restaurant upstairs, the one I wanted to take you to, is closed for renovation and I couldn't get a reservation at the Polo Grill until eight. Is that okay?"

"I guess so," I said reluctantly. I didn't relish the idea of sitting in the bar for another hour. "Does that mean we can't have Beef Wellington and ice cream with hot fudge sauce?" I asked, trying not to whine.

"Actually, the chef that made that stuff died years ago. Probably from high cholesterol. After his death they changed the restaurant to a seafood place. Now they're changing it to something else. I haven't been here in so long, I didn't know. Found out when I called to make the reservations. Sorry about that."

"I'll live," I said, though I wasn't sure I wanted to. I took a big gulp of my martini, shuddering as the ice cold gin seared a path to my stomach. "How did your interviews go?"

"Not bad. A couple of jobs in England sound pretty good, and I could have whichever one I want.

The owners of both companies owed my father big time."

"How nice for you," I said, hiding a sneer. I stuck my swizzle stick through the eyes of two olives and transported them from my glass to my mouth. "Do you think we could get some nuts, or something? I'm starving."

"Sure thing, babe," he said, raising his hand in the air and rudely, but confidently, snapping his fingers. It was a clever trick. The waitress appeared from nowhere, pencil and order pad in hand, smiling from ear to ear. "Bring us a bowl of nuts, honey," he demanded. "And what the hell happened to my drink?"

"Sorry, sir," she replied. "The bartender ran out of Jack Daniels and had to send someone to the storeroom. Your drink will be ready in just a few moments."

"Make it snappy," he said, abruptly turning away from her and facing me. The waitress slunk off toward the bar like a reprimanded poodle. "Now then, where were we?" Ben asked, leaning so close his moist breath hit my cheek.

"You were calling in old debts from your father's old friends."

"No, I mean yesterday, when we were sitting out on the veranda talking about us."

"Us?"

"Yeah. You and me, babe. And how we're finally gonna get it on after all this time. Remember?"

"I remember *you* talking about something like that, but I don't recall giving you any encouragement."

"You accepted my dinner invitation."

"I just wanted to know where my next meal was coming from."

He let out a strained burst of laughter. "You always were quick with a comeback. I like that in a girl."

"I'm not a girl anymore, Ben. I'm all grown up now and I know a line when I hear one. Especially a sloppy one like yours. So why don't you just save the come-ons for somebody else, and let's try to have a pleasant, straightforward evening."

"Ouch! That hurt!"

"I didn't mean it to. I just don't want to spend the rest of the night dodging pointed remarks and sexual innuendoes. You toss them out relentlessly, like a baseball pitching machine."

"Okay! Okay! I get the message. No more lines. No more come-ons. Just plain, straight, *boring* conversation."

"Sounds good to me," I said, smiling.

"So what do you want to talk about? Without sexual innuendoes, I'm at a loss for words." He slouched down in his seat, stretched his legs out under the table and began to sulk.

If I was going to get what I wanted from Ben that night, I realized, I would have to be more straightforward myself. "I want to talk about Jane," I said.

Without a word, Ben jumped to his feet, shot a stormy glance in my direction, and marched across the lounge toward the bar against the back wall. He said something to the bartender, gesturing wildly and angrily with both hands. Then he balled his right hand into a fist and slammed it down on top of the bar, hard.

In shock, the bartender edged away from Ben and said something back, nervously twisting his bar towel into a tight knot. Then he turned toward the mirrored shelves behind him, took down a bottle of bourbon and quickly poured Ben a drink. Ben grabbed the glass and stomped back to our table.

"It's goddamn hard to get a drink around here," he

said, sitting down in a chair on the other side of the table instead of next to me on the banquette. "They still haven't managed to bring any Jack Daniels up from the fucking storeroom. I had to settle for Wild Turkey."

I didn't mention that in light of his current behavior I thought his drink was aptly named. I sat there mutely sipping my martini, studying Ben's face over the rim of my glass and wondering if it was the lack of booze or the mention of Jane that had brought on his violent tantrum. There was only one way to find out.

"Do you have any idea who killed your sister?" I asked him.

He scowled. "Now why the fuck did you have to bring *that* up? I wanted to *forget* about Jane for tonight. I just wanted to focus on *you*, and have some *fun* for a change." He lit up a cigarette, took a deep drag and exhaled angrily.

"Sorry, Ben, but I just *can't* forget about Jane. I found her dead body in the trunk of my car, for God's sake! How do you forget about something like that?"

"I'm sure *I* could think of a way to help you forget," he said with an unmistakable leer. He leaned over and stroked my knee under the table.

"There you go again," I said, crossing my legs and knocking his hand off in the process. "What did you have for lunch today? Testosterone soup?"

As if on cue, the sexy waitress materialized at our table and perkily announced, "Here are your nuts!"

Her perfect timing and inadvertent wordplay were too much for me. I started giggling and I couldn't stop. I felt like I was trapped in a burlesque comedy skit. All that was needed to complete the ridiculous picture was for Spock to jump out from behind the bar with binoculars in one hand and handcuffs in the other.

Though he didn't understand what I was laughing at, Ben started chuckling along with me. He probably thought I was starting to get drunk and have a good time. And I'm sure he was happy that the subject of Jane had been dropped. So happy that he gave the waitress another wink. Then she started giggling, too.

At that point my mirth wore off completely. There I was, drinking and laughing and about to eat a handful of nuts, while Jane was lying six feet under at Nassau Knolls. And sitting right next to me was Jane's callous, oversexed half brother—who, I was beginning to believe, was most likely the demon who had raped and murdered her. I felt heartsick and disgusted and I needed to get away from that table immediately.

"Excuse me please," I said, quickly jumping to my feet. "I have an appointment in the ladies' room."

If there was a restroom near the cocktail lounge, I couldn't find it. I ended up walking down a long marble hallway to a deserted area behind the closed G Club disco. Off to the right was a large ladies' room which was actually two rooms. The first was a lounge as big as my living room.

I stopped there to brush my hair and put on some lipstick before I went into the marble-tiled washroom. I didn't have to use the facilities, but I was in no hurry to get back to my table—or to Ben—so I stalled for time by washing my hands, using some of the hotel's complimentary hand lotion and blotting my lipstick on a tissue I pulled from an engraved silver dispenser.

I was the only one in the ladies' room at the time so I took advantage of the privacy—plus the lavatory's great, echo-like sound effects—and sang a few verses of Patsy Cline's "Crazy" while I tried to get my head straight.

I didn't want to have dinner with Ben anymore. The thought of sharing a meal with him and fending off his advances for another two hours or so made my stomach turn. And it was obvious that he wasn't going to be a willing source of information about Jane's death. Every time I brought the subject up he had a temper fit. I decided that when I got back to the table I would make my excuses—tell him I had a headache or something— and go home.

I had just walked through the door from the lavatory into the lounge when it happened. There was a sudden loud *bam* in back of me—it sounded like the bathroom door had been slammed into the wall—and somebody grabbed me from behind, with one arm around my waist and one hand over my mouth. My bag fell off my shoulder and dropped to the floor as I was lifted off my feet and pulled backward into the corner of the room. Then I was pushed to one side with my back against the wall as Ben stepped in front of me and pinned my wrists to the wall on either side of my head. Before I could scream or utter a single word, he mashed his body into mine and covered my gasping mouth with his own.

Shocked into submission and flooded with adrenalin, I couldn't resist immediately. It took me a few seconds to grasp what was happening and gather enough strength to fight back. Then, by clenching my teeth and jerking my head from side to side, I finally managed to pull my lips away from his.

"You like it like this, don't you, Dixie?" he whispered gruffly, rubbing his hard-on against my hip bone.

"Get away from me or I'll scream."

"Nobody will hear you," he said, breathing hotly

against my neck. "Come on, babe. Loosen up. I booked a suite for us upstairs. Let's forget about our dinner reservation and order room service." He bent his head down and licked the swell of breast just visible above my tube top. Then he trailed his hot wet tongue up the side of my face and stuck it into my left ear.

That did it. My ears are incredibly sensitive and I didn't appreciate having even just one of them violated. I tried to claw Ben's face, but he was holding my wrists so hard to the wall I couldn't do anything but flex my fingers. I tried to push him away with my body but that only turned him on more. In the end, I had to resort to the oldest, most unimaginative, but decidedly most effective method of self-defense known to woman. I bent my right leg and jacked my knee up hard into his overly souped-up nuts.

Grunting and squealing like the pig he had just proved himself to be, Ben jumped back, doubled over, and grabbed hold of his crotch with both hands. I moved away from the wall, took a deep breath, and snatched my purse up from the floor. Then I lunged for the door. Before heading out into the hotel corridor, I took one last look at Ben in the mirror. He was still doubled over and his face had turned kind of purple.

In the corridor, I made a run for it—madly dashing down the deserted marble hallway, past the closed disco, and the Polo Grill Restaurant, and the crowded cocktail lounge area. I didn't slow down until I hit the hotel lobby. The doorman in the green uniform and the green top hat opened the heavy glass door for me and I stepped outside.

It wasn't raining anymore. There was a fragrant mist drifting through the warm night air, blurring the vision and soothing the heart with the promise of spring's renewal. And as I stood there waiting for the valet to bring my car, I couldn't help wondering how Ben would soothe his bruised groin and renew his wounded ego. With a smirk of self-satisfaction, I pictured him limping back into the cocktail lounge and medicating his so-called manhood with countless shots of Wild Turkey.

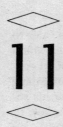

11

I didn't even wait until I got home. About halfway to my house I pulled into a Taco Bell, jumped out of the car, and popped into the public phone booth just outside the well-lit entrance. I got the number of the Garden City Hotel from Information and called it. After speaking to the hotel operator, and then the bartender, I managed to get the redheaded waitress on the line.

"You waited on me in the cocktail lounge earlier this evening," I told her. "I ordered a martini with five olives. Remember?"

"Yeah?" she said.

"I was sitting with a big guy with long hair, a mustache, and an earring."

"Yeah?"

"Is he still there by any chance?"

"Sure is. You wanna talk to him?"

"No!" I said quickly. "I just want to talk to *you* for a second. I know this'll sound crazy, but I'm calling to warn you to watch out for that guy. He booked a room in the hotel tonight, and I have the feeling he might hang out till you get off work and try to get you to spend the night there with him."

"So what if he does?"

"Well, I just wanted to tell you to stay away from him. He's a dangerous man."

"Oh yeah?"

I recognized the attitude and the tone of voice. She thought I was a rejected girlfriend, wild with jealousy and looking for revenge. She thought I was trying to hurt her chances for an exciting new relationship with a gorgeous rich guy. "You don't understand," I told her. "I'm telling you the truth. He really *is* dangerous."

"Well, you don't have to worry about me, *ma'am*," she said, letting me know that, in comparison with her, I was just an old bag. "I can take care of myself."

I was tempted to hang up and let her find out if she could, but the thought of a naked, pale-skinned, red-headed corpse being discovered in an unsuspecting hotel guest's car trunk was more than I could bear.

"Listen to me carefully, young lady," I said, using my most authoritative tone. "This is Detective Sergeant Annie March speaking. Nassau County Police Department. Homicide. This is no joke. I'm calling to let you know that the man who's been making eyes at you all night, the man who's probably snapping his fingers for you to come to his table *right now*, is the primary suspect in a rape and murder case under current investigation."

"Oh my God!"

"Don't flirt with him. Don't encourage his advances. Don't give him your name, address, or phone number. And don't, under any circumstances, go up to his room with him."

"Oh, I won't! I won't!" she cried.

"And if you see him coming on to any other women in the lounge, please find a way to warn them against him. It could be a matter of life and death."

"Oh, I will!"

"Thank you for your help and cooperation," I said. "Have a pleasant evening and take care of yourself." I hung up before she could ask me any questions.

Oh, great! I said to myself. *Tampering with evidence, dangerous and reckless driving, and now impersonating an officer. How many crimes am I going to commit trying to prove I'm not a criminal?*

Before returning to the car, I went inside the Bell and bought two Taco Supremes and a Burrito Grande to go. Then I got back behind the wheel, shoved Bonnie Raitt's *Nick of Time* album into the tape deck and headed for home with "Thing Called Love" turned loud enough to rock my soul and silence my mind.

As I pulled into my driveway I noticed a strange car parked on the street in front of my house, just out of range of the nearest streetlight. I gathered up my stuff, got out of my car, and locked it, staring at the strange vehicle the whole time. I couldn't tell if it was occupied or not. But after a few seconds of peering through the darkness, my eyes adjusted to the lack of light and I was able to perceive the color and the make of the car. It was a dark blue Chevy. The same one that had been following me that afternoon. I decided to go over and introduce myself to Detective Spockett if he was there.

There was a man in the car, but it wasn't Spock. It was Eddie. And he was sound asleep, slouched down in the driver's seat with his head resting against the frame of the half-open window. I wanted to reach inside and stroke his friendly unshaven face, but I didn't. I knocked on the window instead.

"Huh?" he muttered, jerking his head away from the door and pulling his body to an upright position. His eyes were open but they weren't in focus yet.

"Gotcha!" I said with a grin. "I suspected you boys were sleeping on the job, and now I know for sure."

"Oh!" he said, suddenly realizing where he was and who was talking to him. "You okay, Annie? I've been waiting here a long time." He rubbed his face and his eyes with both hands.

"Sure I'm okay," I said. "I'm just hungry. Come on inside and share my elegant dinner." I held the Taco Bell bag up toward the window and wiggled it.

Eddie got out of the car and followed me into the house. "Where have you been all evening?" he asked after we had settled down at the kitchen table and divvied up the food. "I was worried about you."

"I had dinner with a friend," I said, almost choking on the word *friend*.

"Then how come you're so hungry?" He took a big bite of his taco and stared at my face while he chewed.

I was caught up short on that one, so I quickly bit into my half of the burrito. The etiquette of not talking with a full mouth gave me ample time to think up an answer. "I didn't like what I ordered," I said when I'd swallowed. "Meat loaf. The menu said it was ground round, but it tasted like ground hound."

Eddie laughed and poured himself a glass of Sprite from the bottle I had put out on the table. Then he looked me straight in the eye and asked, "And where did you spend the afternoon?"

Since I knew that Spock, and therefore Eddie, knew exactly where I had been that day, I figured I'd better stick as close to the truth as possible. "I went out to Sands Point to visit Mrs. Masterson. She looked so devastated at the funeral I thought I would try to console her.

"The murder of a loved one is impossible to accept," I told him. "I know from experience. After my husband was killed, I lived in a daze of denial for months. The horror of it still astounds me."

Eddie put down his drink and gazed at me with obvious compassion. "It must have been tough losing your husband like that," he said.

"The toughest."

"I'm sorry."

"Thanks."

"I didn't say anything that first night, when you told me about the way he died, because I had to focus my attention on the Masterson killing. I hope I didn't appear insensitive."

"Not at all."

He gave me a grateful smile and then took a sip of his drink. "How long did you stay at the Masterson estate?" he asked, getting back to the murder at hand.

"A couple of hours. I had a long talk with Bette and then took a walk with Daisy. Afterward, I went into Port Washington to visit my father. He still lives there, in an apartment near the house our family used to own."

"I see," Eddie said, nodding. He believed I was telling the truth and, in a way, I was. I was just leaving out a couple of little details—like the *real* reasons I went to both of those places.

"Was Ben there?" Eddie asked me.

"Why would Ben be at my father's apartment?"

Eddie rolled his eyes. "You know what I mean."

He was right. I did know. And I was acting a little too coy for my own good. "Ben wasn't home." I answered quickly. "His stepmother said he had some business appointments in Manhattan."

"Hmmm . . ." Eddie mused, staring at the tabletop with a serious look on his face. He finished off his taco and started in on his half of the burrito.

"How's everything at home?" I jumped in, anxious to change the subject while I had the chance.

"Okay," he said, but he didn't look like he meant it.

"Your wife must be glad to be back in her own house."

"She'd rather be in Florida."

"What?"

"Florida," he repeated. "For some reason she's gotten it into her head she wants to move down there. Last year it was California. The year before that it was Paris. This year it's Florida. She wants me to apply to the Homicide Department in Ft. Lauderdale."

"Are you going to do it?" I asked, holding my breath. The thought of Eddie moving away made my head hurt. Even if I couldn't have him for myself, I felt happier and safer with him nearby.

"No," he insisted. "I hate rednecks and I hate the sun. I'd rather work in a coal mine. Besides, even if we *did* move down there, she'd be itching to move again in a year or so. That's just the way Claudine is. Everything is always better somewhere else." And the way he said it made me wonder if Claudine had ever hinted that husbands might be better somewhere else, too.

He looked so depressed I changed the subject again. "So how's the case going?" I asked, slipping into my self-restrained, innocent little bystander mode. "Turn up any new leads?"

"Maybe," he said. His eyes stopped brooding and started to twinkle.

"What is it? What did you find out?"

"Oh, a few things, actually."

"Like what?"

"Like where the murder probably occurred."

"Really? Where? How did you find out? Tell me everything!" My placid composure became a distant memory. I was as restrained as a fox terrier with a fresh meaty bone. "What else did you learn? How many people have you questioned? Do you have any suspects?"

"Whoa!" Eddie said, holding his hands up to stop my barrage. "Cool down! You know I can't answer those questions, Annie."

"Why?"

"Because you're still under investigation yourself. Because I'm not allowed to discuss the details of the case with anybody outside of the department. Because I don't want you to become any more involved than you already are."

"Then why did you tell me anything in the first place?" I whined.

"I wanted you to know that we're working very hard on this case. And we're making very good progress," he said. "You may think we're not doing our job, but you're wrong. Nassau County has the best Homicide department in the state. We'll get this murderer and we'll get him soon. You don't have to worry about that. We don't miss a trick."

"That's very comforting," I said. I thought about the Filofax hidden behind the sweatshirts on my closet shelf and wondered if Eddie would consider that a missed trick.

"Gotta run," he said, rising to his feet and retrieving

the trench coat slung over the back of his chair. "Miles to go before I sleep."

"Unless you can grab another nap in the car."

He smiled. "Nope. I'm driving the department's best undercover car and Spock wants to use it tonight. If I'm gonna do any more snoring on the job I'd better wait till I get back to the office." He smiled again. Then I followed him through the living room to the front door.

"Be careful," I said, suddenly overcome with the fear that must plague every policeman's wife. My own near-escape from bodily harm earlier in the evening had made me particularly sensitive to the idea of danger. "Don't try to push around anybody bigger than you are."

"Nothing to worry about tonight," he said. "I won't be pushing anything but a pencil." He opened the door and started to go through it, but suddenly turned back to face me again. "*You're* the one who needs to be careful, Annie," he said, putting his hands on my shoulders and staring into my eyes with an imploring look. "Please make sure that you are." Then, quick as a whisper, he raised his right hand and brushed the tips of his fingers down my face.

Several moments after Eddie left my house and drove away, I was still standing at my open front door, peering out into the black velvet night like a dreamy schoolgirl. A thousand tiny fires were burning on my cheek.

Just as I came to my senses and decided to lock up for the night, Philly's little red Sundance pulled into my driveway and screeched to a stop right behind my little black Shadow. Philly jumped out of the car and ran up to my front porch, her bright orange slicker slapping against her body like a rubber choir robe.

"Where the dickens you been, girl? I been callin' and callin' and gettin' no answer all evenin' and all night! Woodrow's out of town on business and I been sittin' there in the 'partment, all by myself, dialin' the phone over and over again like a numskull. I was so worried 'bout you I couldn't stand it another minute. I had to get dressed and drive on over here to satisfy myself that you were all right." She stamped her feet and angrily scraped the soles of her shiny purple ankle boots against the slate porch floor.

"I thought I was gonna find you lyin' in the middle of the floor with a bullet in the middle of your brain," she went on, "and here you are standin' big as you please in a wide-open door lookin' up at the stars like a darn fool! I don't know what to do 'bout you, Annie. You got to have your head examined 'fore somebody shoots it off."

"Take it easy, Philly!" I cried. "I'm fine! I really am. How can I convince you that everything's okay?"

"Well you can start by takin' your fool self into the house and closin' the damn door!" she sputtered, casting wild glances around the yard like a child looking for monsters. "And you can take me with you."

Inside, Philly took off her slicker and hung it on the coatrack. She was wearing her nursing uniform.

"You really *did* come prepared for an emergency," I teased. Philly loved bright colors and would never wear her uniform, or *anything* that was all white, unless she had to.

"I was so out of whack I put on the first thing I could find," she explained, "and this was sitting on a chair right by the bed."

"Good," I said. "Since you've got your uniform with you, you can spend the night and go to work straight from here in the morning."

"Huh . . . ? Well, yeah, I guess I could," she said, warming to the idea. "That way I could keep a eye on you. Make sure you don't go runnin' off in the middle of the night to some back alley or crack house lookin' for your precious killer!"

"Oh, come on, Philly! It's not like that and you know it. I'm too much of a chicken to put myself in any real danger. I'm just poking around a little bit, seeing if I can find out anything to help the cops. Stop worrying about me."

"I'll stop worryin' when you stop pokin'."

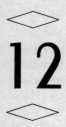

12

I changed into my gray sweatpants and my Rolling Stones stuck-out-tongue T-shirt and gave Philly a pair of hot pink pajamas. She was happy that the color matched her nail polish. I made a huge bowl of popcorn, sprinkled it with garlic salt, grabbed a couple of beers, and lugged the whole mess out to the coffee table in the living room. Curled up on separate couches, we guzzled Budweiser, stuffed our faces and talked until two in the morning.

In spite of her anguish over my safety, Philly was anxious to hear what I had learned about the case that day. I told her all about going out to the Masterson estate, talking with Bette and Daisy, and being tailed by Spock. I told her what Daisy had said about Ben and then I described my meeting with him at the Garden City Hotel. I *didn't* tell her about what happened in the ladies' room. I didn't want another lecture about how I was "fixin'" to get myself killed.

"Did you tell Frecklepuss 'bout all this?" she asked me.

"No. I don't want him to know what I'm doing."

"Why?"

"Because he'll try to make me stop. He's as worried about me as you are. Also, the other detectives he works with still think I had something to do with the murder. And the more involved I get, the guiltier I look. He's afraid for me on both ends."

"A man after my own heart."

"The cops think they know where Jane was killed," I told her, "but Eddie, uh, I mean Sergeant Lincoln, wouldn't give me any of the details."

"No reason to talk fancy with me, girlfriend. Call him Eddie if you want to. I know you've got the hots for him."

"Well, it doesn't matter *what* I've got for him. He's a married man. Has two kids, too."

"That's too bad," Philly said. "I was hopin' you two would get it on. This is the first time I've ever seen you warm up for a guy."

"Is it that obvious?"

"As plain as your face."

"You mean the *nose* on my face," I said, automatically falling into my tutor role.

"I said what I meant, honey!" Philly gave me a goofy look and started laughing. She snickered and giggled until I finally got the joke and laughed along with her.

"So Frecklepuss knows where Goldilocks was killed, but he won't tell you?" she asked.

"Right. But I don't really care because I think I know anyway."

"Really? Where?"

"Well I can't be sure, of course, but from my own observations, and from what I heard at the police department, I'd say it happened out at the Masterson estate. Maybe in one of the flower gardens, but probably in the greenhouse."

"What makes you think that?"

"Remember the conversation I told you about? The one I overheard while I was sitting in Lieutenant O'Donnell's office?"

"Yeah. That's how you found out the girl was raped."

"Right. But I found out some other stuff, too. The two cops who were talking about the forensic report said the only clothes found with the body were a pair of sweatpants, a T-shirt, socks, and a pair of panties. No bra and no shoes. I don't think Jane would have gone *out* dressed like that, so unless she was kidnapped or something, she must have been at home when it happened.

"Also," I continued, "the cops said mica flecks, sand, humus, and traces of manure—all ingredients of potting soil—were found on her clothes and in her hair. And there was dirt embedded in the knees of her sweatpants. I found out from Daisy that Jane was an avid gardener, so it seems possible that she was raped, or shot, or both, while working in the garden or the greenhouse. My money's on the greenhouse because she was killed between 7 and 8 P.M., and I don't think she would have been working out in the garden after dark."

"'Sides that," Philly said, "any rapist or murderer would rather jump somebody *inside* a buildin', 'specially a empty buildin'."

"Right! It would cut the risk of being seen or heard. And the Masterson greenhouse is quite far away from the main house, so the chances of anyone inside the house seeing or hearing anything would be pretty slim. I asked Daisy if she noticed anything strange that night, but she said no. She didn't hear any screaming or shooting. She thought Jane spent the evening in her room and then died in her sleep."

"How 'bout that gardener man?" Philly asked. "You said he has a room attached to the greenhouse. Wouldn't he have heard somethin'?"

"If he was there, he would. But he was probably home with the wife and kiddies that night." I was just supposing, I realized, so I made a mental note to ask Juan a few questions the next time I went out to the Masterson estate.

"How 'bout Goldilocks's mama? Wouldn't she know if her daughter was home or not?"

"Negative. Bette Masterson is riddled with cancer. She takes a bucketful of sleeping pills and painkillers and goes to bed early. She wouldn't know where *any-body* was, including herself."

"Was Big Ben home that evenin'? Did you ask him if he heard anything or if he knew where his sister was?"

"He told the cops he thought she was out on a date. But he told *me* that Jane was in love with and having a mad affair with her doctor, Niles Stanwyck. And if that's true, it seems kind of unlikely that she would have been out on a date with somebody else. From what I can tell, she didn't have many friends at all. There were no peo-ple her own age at the funeral, and there are hardly any names or phone numbers written down in her Filofax. Dr. Stanwyck is the only personal listing."

"So maybe she was out with the doc."

"It's possible, I guess, but I don't think so. Would she wear a T-shirt and dirty sweatpants to meet her lover? Besides, Ben said Jane and Niles usually met in his office—during office hours—and conducted their love-making on his office couch. So Niles was probably try-ing to keep the affair secret. I don't think he would have

taken Jane out in public. Nina Stanwyck strikes me as
the kind of wife who keeps her husband on a very short
leash."

Philly finished her beer and squeezed the empty can
into the shape of an hourglass. "So you think Big Ben
was lyin' 'bout Goldilocks bein' out on a date?"

"Lying through his perfectly capped teeth."

"Gracious!" Philly cried. "Sounds to me like you got
your mind made up who the murderer is!"

"My mind's not made up, but it sure is full of suspicion."

"You really think your high school boyfriend raped
and murdered his own *sister?*"

"Half sister," I corrected, "and he *wasn't* my
boyfriend! But, yes, I'm beginning to think Ben did it."
I got up off the couch, grabbed the empty popcorn bowl
and beer cans and headed for the kitchen.

"Where the heck you goin', girl?" Philly shrieked.
"You can't pop a zinger like that and then walk right out
the room! You gonna just leave me hangin' here like a
string of snot?"

"I'll be right back," I said, laughing. "I just want to
get some more beer." I tossed the empty cans in the
recycling bin, put the bowl in the sink, and took two
more Buds out of the refrigerator.

"How come you think it was Ben?" Philly asked as
soon as I returned to the living room. She was sitting
stick straight on the edge of the couch. Her wildly
blinking eyes and scruffy blond hair gave her the look of
a little girl who'd just woken up from a nightmare.

"Well, as far as I can tell, he's the only one who stood
to gain by Jane's death. He's the only one with a
motive."

"Motive? What motive?"

"Money, of course. With Jane out of the way, Ben will probably inherit the entire family estate when his stepmother dies. And given Bette Masterson's current physical condition, he shouldn't have long to wait."

I sat down and outlined my theory to Philly. "I think when Ben first found out his stepmother had cancer, he got a divorce. He didn't want to have to split his inheritance with his wife. Then, when he heard that Bette had gotten very sick and might be close to death, he high-tailed it back to Sands Point with one thought in mind: Jane had to die *before* Bette. Otherwise, half of everything might go to his half sister. And maybe Ben just never learned how to share."

Philly stared into the center of the room for a few moments and then began nodding her head. "Makes sense, girl, makes sense," she said. "I get what you're sayin' and I can buy most of your story. It fits like a baby in a belly. 'Cept for one thing—"

"What's that?"

"The *rape*," she insisted. "Are you sayin' he raped her, too? 'Cause if you are, I won't believe *that*. What kind of man would rape his own sister?"

"The lousy kind," I said. "The same kind who would *kill* his own sister. And where have you been anyway? Off in the Yukon somewhere? Don't you watch the news anymore? Or *Hard Copy*? Or *Geraldo*? Incestuous rape is the hottest new fad since bungee jumping. *Everybody's* doing it."

Philly screwed her face up into a grimace of disgust. "They oughta line every last one of 'em up against a wall and shoot their sticky dicks off."

"I'm with you, kid."

Then a new idea suddenly took root in my brain, growing quickly and sprouting branches. "I just thought of something else," I told Philly. "Maybe Ben hired a *hit man* to kill Jane. That could explain everything. Maybe the hit man was one of those sicker-than-sick psychos who gets sexually turned on when he's about to kill somebody. So, when he saw that his mark was a beautiful young blond with a drop-dead gorgeous body, he decided to rape her before he shot her."

"Yeeuck!"

"Ditto."

"Sounds plausible, though," Philly said, using one of the big fat show-off words I had taught her. "And I can believe *that* notion easier than I can believe the other one."

"Hmmm, maybe. But whoever actually pulled the trigger, there's still one other thing I can't figure out," I said, uncurling my legs and propping my feet on the edge of the coffee table.

"What's that, Sherlock?"

"How the hell did Jane's body wind up in the trunk of *my* car? And, more importantly, *why?*"

"Maybe your old boyfriend was tryin' to tell you somethin'."

"*Stop* calling him my boyfriend!"

"Okay! Okay!" Philly said, holding her pink-taloned hands up in surrender. "I just said that 'cause it sounds like he had a big crush on you back in high school. And I can't help wonderin' if maybe he's still hurt 'bout the way you treated him. Maybe he decided to put the body—or have his hit man put the body—in your trunk just to get even."

"The way I treated him? I didn't *do* anything for him to be hurt about!" I cried. *Not back then, anyway*, I thought with a secret smile.

"Then maybe he just *thinks* you did. You know, like

maybe he was comin' on to you in class one day, and you weren't payin' him any mind, so he thought you were disrespectin' him or somethin'. Maybe you broke his heart and never even knew it. And maybe it hurt so bad he never got over it."

"That's impossible! We barely knew each other."

"Now it's *my* turn to ask where *you* been!" Philly said. "Since when does a person have to *know* another person to get witched by them? Haven't you watched the news lately? Seems like every day there's another story 'bout somebody gettin' raped or killed by some nut job who got himself all worked up into one of them fatal attraction-type deals. Oprah had a show on it just last week. It's the hottest new fad since rap dancin'!"

"Touché," I said with a snarl.

"Don't mention it," Philly purred.

I wanted to ignore her theory, but I couldn't. Everything she said was just too damn *possible*. So I found myself doing some heavy-duty wondering. I wondered about some of the things Ben had said to me on the porch after the funeral. I wondered about the fact that he'd known my husband had been murdered. I wondered why he'd never shown surprise over, or even *mentioned,* the incredible coincidence that *I* had been the one to discover Jane's body. Suddenly, Philly's suggestion didn't seem farfetched at all. For one schizophrenic second I even wondered if Ben could have been the one who had killed *Sam*.

I shivered. I couldn't bear to think about it anymore. Then a wave of exhaustion swept over me. I stretched my arms over my head and twisted my neck to get the kinks out. "Well, there's no way we can solve this case tonight," I said, "so we might as well hit the sack. What time do you have to get up in the morning?"

"'Bout five-thirty."

"Ugh. You'll only get three and a half hours of sleep," I said, feeling guilty that worrying over me had robbed Philly of a peaceful night. I knew how hard she worked and how much she needed her rest.

"Yeah. My fanny'll be draggin' on the floor tomorrow. And Woodrow's comin' back so I'll have to get to the grocery and make a big dinner when I get home." She stood up and slowly shuffled into the hallway leading to the guest bedroom.

"That won't leave you much time to work on your reading and your homework assignments," I said, following her and stopping at the door to my own bedroom. "Do you want to cancel Thursday's lesson?"

"No way, girlfriend! My mind's a terrible thing to waste!" Smiling, she turned toward me and pushed her glasses higher on her nose with one long brown finger. Then she focused all of her concentration on my face. "What's the matter, honey?" she asked. "You 'fraid to go back to the library?"

I *did* feel uneasy about something, so I took a few seconds to think about her question. "No," I eventually answered. "There's no reason to fear the library more than any other place. If Ben really is after me in some way, then he can nail me *anywhere*. He must know where I live, where I shop, what gym I go to—"

"Annie, *please* forget 'bout all this fool detective business!" Philly begged. "Come stay with Woodrow and me."

"Thanks for the invite," I said. "I'll think about it. But not right now! Right now I'm going to get into my bed, pull the covers over my head, and snooze like a cat for the rest of the night. There's not that much of it left."

"Okay, babe," Philly said, opening the door of the

guest room. "Sweet dreams!" she called out as she went inside.

Minutes later, as I closed my eyes and burrowed my head into the pillow, I wondered if my dreams would ever be sweet again.

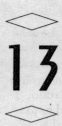

13

When I woke up the next morning Philly was gone. She had, in fact, already been at work for three hours. Her bed was made and the hot pink pajamas I had loaned her were sitting, neatly folded, on top. When I went into the kitchen to make a pot of coffee I found the note she left me: *Thanks Annie. See you tomorow. Pack a sootcase. You will come home with me after the lesson.*

The carefully printed message filled me with pride. Four years ago she couldn't have written it. I smiled at the misspellings and decided to take the note with me on Thursday so we could study those words together. I would *not*, however, take a suitcase.

After spending most of the night worrying that Ben might be trying to get even with me for something that happened in the past, or, even worse, that he might try to get revenge for what had more recently happened in the hotel ladies' room, I had come to the conclusion that running scared and hiding out would only prolong the problem.

The sooner Ben was behind bars, the sooner I would feel safe again. And, I figured, the sooner I could find out the truth about Jane's death, the sooner Ben would be arrested.

I would continue my personal investigation, I decided, but I would also do everything I could to protect myself in the process. So the minute I finished my first cup of coffee, I got on the phone and made next-day appointments to have an alarm system installed in my house and deadbolt locks put on all the doors.

As I was making myself a breakfast of whole wheat toast and chunky peanut butter, the phone rang. I licked the peanut butter off the knife and answered it.

"At last!" said the shrill, nasal voice on the other end. "If you don't get yourself an answering machine soon, I'm buying you one for your birthday." It was Ellen Drucker, a woman I had worked with years ago, when we were both right out of college and beginning our publishing careers with entry level jobs on a teen magazine. Ellen was an associate editor for *Glamour* now.

"Hi Ellen," I said. "Long time no talk."

"Well it's not because I haven't *tried*. I've been calling you every hour on the hour for two whole days!"

"Why? What's up?"

"I need a good feature story and I need it *fast*. I just got back to work after a two-month leave of absence— *with* pay—and my beloved coworkers are still so jealous and pissed off about it they're making my life hell," she said, talking a mile a minute in her usual flippant and nasty way. "At the editorial meeting on Monday, Sheila Shithead Cramer suggested that—since I'm so well-rested and, no doubt, *dying* to get busy again—*I* should be responsible for conceiving, assigning, and editing next issue's lead article. That bitch! Thanks to her I have to come up with a great idea and submit a smashing cover line for approval *tomorrow*. And my brain is still baking on the beach in Acapulco! You've got to help me, Annie. I'm desperate!"

"When do you need the article?"

"A week from this Friday. The next Monday at the latest."

I groaned. With everything that was happening in my life, I really didn't feel like adding an urgent deadline to the stew. "Don't you have anything in your files?" I asked her.

"Well, to be honest with you, I let my files get kind of low. I was so preoccupied with buying the right clothes and accessories for my trip that I just sort of lost track of things at work. I had to shop for three new bathing suits and you know how hard *that* is."

"Well, I'm kind of preoccupied myself right now, Ellen. Couldn't you find somebody else?"

"Please, Annie! You're the only one I can count on. You're the only one I know who can work fast enough to get this assignment in on time. You always turn in clean copy, too. You've got to help me!"

"Oh, okay," I said, sighing loudly. "What do you want the story to be on? Have you given it any thought at all?"

"A little," she mumbled unconvincingly. "Shit! Where did I put my notes?" I could hear her banging books and flapping papers around on top of her desk. When we had worked together at *Teen Stars*, Ellen's desk always looked (and occasionally smelled) like the Staten Island landfill. "Oh, I'm such a wreck," she moaned, "I can't find anything today!"

"Never mind," I said quickly. "I've got an idea."

"What?" she gasped.

"Plastic surgery. With the focus on the body instead of the face. Breast implants, liposuction, tummy tucks—stuff like that."

"Oh, that's no good, Annie," she said sadly. "It's too much work. You'd have to do a lot of research and interview at least one well-known, respectable surgeon. There isn't enough time for all of that."

"Maybe there is. I met a plastic surgeon just last Monday. And he's obviously successful. Sands Point house, Mercedes, the whole bit. Looks like the type who'd like to have some national publicity, too. I'm sure I could talk to him. Maybe today, even."

"Really? That would be great! I'd look like a real hustler if I could bring in something like that. Let's do it! Get on it right away. But what'll we call it? I've got to submit the title tomorrow and it's got to be good. How about 'The Cutting Edge'?"

"Too cute and confusing. Something simple would be better. Something like 'The Perfect Body'."

"That's it!" she cried. "'The Perfect Body.' I'll give it a catchy subtitle and it'll be *perfect!*"

"Good," I said. "I'll try to see the surgeon today and get back to you soon."

"You've really saved my life, Annie. How can I ever thank you?"

"Just promise you *won't* buy me an answering machine," I told her. "I hate the damn things."

The local map I had borrowed from my father's apartment got me to the Stanwyck residence without a single wrong turn. I pulled into the long straight driveway, drove across the well-tended but almost treeless acre fronting the immense ultra-modern house, and parked my car in a stone-paved area to the side of the main entrance. As I got out of my car I saw a flight of steps leading from the parking site down to another entrance on the lower level. Dr. Stanwyck's office maybe? I couldn't be sure, so I decided to try the front door first.

In spite of all the time I'd spent in Sands Point over the last couple of days, I still felt out of place here. Like a seashell in the desert. My blue jeans and black turtleneck were from The Gap instead of one of the glitzy designer shops at the Americana shopping center. My clear fingernails had been cut, filed, and lacquered at home instead of in a high-priced beauty salon. My blazer was made of wool instead of cashmere and my cowboy boots were leather, not lizard.

The petite dark-haired maid who cracked open the door seemed to take all of this into account. When I asked if either Dr. or Mrs. Stanwyck were at home, she looked me over from head to toe and then stood there for a second with an "I smell excrement" expression on her face—wondering, no doubt, if she should bother her classy employers with the lowly likes of me.

"Who are you and what do you want?" she demanded, baring her small, even teeth in a threatening sneer. I wondered why there was no Beware Of Dog sign posted in the yard.

"My name is Annie March," I told her. "I met the Stanwycks last Monday at the Masterson funeral. I'm a writer for *Glamour* magazine."

I'll never understand why people get excited when they hear you work for a magazine, but they often do. And the maid's sudden arousal was obvious. Her eyes grew as big as coat buttons and she gave me a broad, simpering smile. She even batted her eyelashes a few times. Maybe she always dreamed of becoming a model while she mopped the floors.

"Come in, please," she said, opening the door wide enough for me to enter. "Dr. Stanwyck is unavailable. I'll tell Mrs. Stanwyck you're here." As she turned and walked toward an expansive hallway on the right, she tossed another smile over her shoulder like a flirtatious hooker.

After she left I stood stiffly in the huge, high-ceilinged entrance hall. The inside of the house looked a lot like the outside: colossal and white with towering walls of glass; accents of marble and metal; all straight lines and sharp angles. A shaft of sun shot through the prominent hall skylight and struck the top of my head, making my hair hot. I moved out of the solar beam and started snooping around, checking out the decor and art work.

The walls featured three large pastel abstracts and several signed and numbered black and white prints that looked like Rorschach ink blots. A white marble table topped with a tall vase of pink silk flowers stood against the far wall. In the very center of the hall, a plush round white rug floated on the floor like a cloud. As mindful of dirty footprints as any woman who's used to cleaning her own house, I walked *around* it instead of *on* it.

I was about to creep around the corner and sneak a peek into the living room when the maid returned. "Mrs. Stanwyck will see you in the dining room," she said, smoothing the skirt of her pink and gray uniform and batting her eyelashes again. "Follow me, please."

I trailed the maid down the hall, wondering what Nina was doing in the dining room. It was just eleven forty-five, not really lunchtime yet. Maybe she'd overslept, I speculated, and was having a late breakfast. I hoped that was the case. Good manners would dictate that she offer me something to eat, too, and I was getting hungry again.

But there wasn't any food on the table. There was just a giant, partially done jigsaw puzzle with hundreds, maybe thousands of unattached pieces, all sorted into different piles by color. Hunched over the puzzle like a miser over money, Nina Stanwyck sat at the near side of the long dining table with her back to the dining room door. She didn't look up when we walked in.

After a few seconds of awkward silence, the maid cleared her throat and said, "Mrs. March is here, Miss."

"Oh!" Nina exclaimed, jerking to an upright position as if suddenly awakened from a dream. When she turned to face me I saw that the flesh around her eyes was dark and puffy and her pupils were glazed.

Without the turban she didn't look like Marlene Dietrich anymore. She was still beautiful, though. Heavy waves of honey-blond hair fell to her shoulders, framing her face with an eerie golden glow. Even in the bright sunlight—plenty of which streamed through the tall dining room windows—her skin looked flawless. Thick brown lashes rimmed her sea green eyes and coral lipstick emphasized the exotic shape of her plump, wide mouth. She wore a peach-colored sweater unbuttoned at the throat, a gold braid necklace, and a softly tailored pair of beige pants—cashmere, of course.

"Hello, Mrs. March," she said, grabbing onto the edge of the table and slowly pulling herself to a standing position. She tottered slightly, like a frail old woman—or a younger one with a bad hangover. I wondered if she'd been hitting the Chivas again. "It's Annie, isn't it?" she asked, smiling weakly.

"That's right," I said. "And you're Nina?" She was at

least seven years younger than I. Rich lady or not, there was no way I was going to call her Mrs. Stanwyck.

"Uh, yes . . . Nina," she stammered, as if she had, for a moment, forgotten her own name. "Please have a seat," she said, indicating an ivory-colored ladder-back chair across the table from her own.

The cold shrew I had met the afternoon of Jane's funeral was gone. In her place was a polite phantom. Nina Stanwyck was either sick, or exhausted, or on her best behavior. "What can I do for you?" she inquired as we both sat down.

"Well, it's really your husband I came to see," I told her. "I'm writing an article about cosmetic surgery for *Glamour* magazine and I was hoping he would give me an interview."

"My husband? An interview?"

"Yes. When I accepted the assignment, I recalled meeting you and your husband after Jane Masterson's funeral, and I remembered that he had been Jane's plastic surgeon." I didn't know what to say, exactly, so I just let my mouth flap along. "I was hoping Dr. Stanwyck could meet with me soon to discuss the different kinds of operations he performs—what the various benefits, risks, and costs might be. A recent poll proves our readers are very interested in cosmetic surgery. And, since the article I'm working on is going to be the lead cover feature, I thought—"

"I doubt it," she interrupted. Her voice was as faint as a baby's sigh.

"Excuse me?"

"I doubt it," she repeated, gazing down at the jigsaw puzzle and moving a few of the blue pieces around with her index finger. "I can't answer for my husband, of course, but I don't think he'll want to do your interview."

"Why?" I asked, trying not to sound too anxious. Suddenly I was as nervous about getting that damn article done as I was about finding Jane's killer. Then I chided myself. Little Miss Conscientious. Why should I be more concerned about Ellen's job security than she had been herself?

"Jane Masterson's death was a horrible shock to Niles," Nina explained with a dainty shudder. "He hasn't gotten over it yet. He hasn't gone to his clinic in Manhattan—or even into his office downstairs—since it happened." She continued to stare at the pile of blue puzzle pieces.

"I'm very sorry to hear that," I said, pretending total ignorance of the situation. "Was your husband a friend of Jane's as well as her doctor?"

"You could say that, I guess, but it would only be a half-truth. The whole truth is that they were lovers. Aha!" she suddenly cried, her pale face lighting up like a signal flare. "*There's* the little rascal I've been looking for!" She picked up a single jigsaw piece from the pile and fitted it to one segment of the assembled puzzle. As she gingerly tapped it into place, her coral mouth curled into a jubilant smile.

I was startled into silence by Nina's offhand admission. So she *did* know that Niles had been sleeping with Jane. What's more, she didn't seem to give a damn.

"I can see that I've shocked you," she said, looking up from the puzzle and gazing intently into my eyes. "I guess I *do* sound hard-hearted or something. It's just that it's been going on for so long. Jane Masterson wasn't the first. She was more like the fifteenth. Poor Niles. He just can't help himself. He's a sucker for a pretty face—even if he has to make the face pretty himself."

"You don't seem to be too upset about it," I ventured.

"I'm not. One gets used to things, you know? He'll have a new lover before long, and I just hope she's good to him. When he's happy, I'm happy," she said, looking as if she really meant it. "But you didn't come here to talk about *me*," she added, pulling herself to her feet again. "You want to talk to Niles, and I think he's in the library. Come, I'll take you to him."

We walked down a long wide hall to the right, past a sunlit breakfast room and a dazzling stainless steel kitchen, into another hallway, past a small sitting room, through a glass-walled conservatory and, finally, into the library.

But why they called it the library was a mystery to me. There were no books there at all. Not even a dictionary. There were lots of book*shelves*—great, soaring, floor-to-ceiling and wall-to-wall stacks of shelves—but they were all full of pottery and sculpture. Modern stuff, mostly. Oddly formed glass objects, brightly colored ceramic pieces, and glossy silver things shaped like circles, squares, and pyramids. Blinding rays of sun poured through the glass wall on the left and reflected off the numerous shiny surfaces in the room, bouncing in all directions. I wished I had on my sunglasses.

Niles Stanwyck sat slumped in a white leather chair near the white marble fireplace with his legs stretched out on a white leather ottoman. His eyes were closed and his chin was resting on his chest.

"Niles, dear," Nina said, leading me into the center of the mauve carpet. "Look who's here. It's Annie March. Ben Masterson's friend. The one he introduced us to last Monday? She wants to talk to you about doing a magazine interview."

If Niles had been sleeping, he wasn't anymore. He opened his big blue eyes and looked up at me with unconcealed curiosity. "What magazine?" he asked, sitting up straight in his chair and putting his feet on the floor. Not a single "hello" or "how are you?" was offered. His social graces were as underdeveloped as his maid's.

"I write for *Glamour*," I told him, deciding to skip over the polite preliminaries myself. "I'm doing an article on cosmetic surgery—the lead cover story for the next issue—and I was hoping to get some quotes from you. The article will focus on body work rather than facelifts, and you will be the only surgeon interviewed. The magazine will give you exclusive credit and full copy approval."

"I think you should do it, Niles," his wife interjected. "It would help you get your mind off things."

"It would also make you famous," I jumped back in, going straight for the jugular. "*Glamour* has a national circulation of one and a half million. With the international circulation, you're up to two. Our readership is mostly female, so that's *two million women* we're talking about. I don't have to tell you what that kind of exposure could do for your business, I mean practice."

I had him and I knew it. One look at his face told me he was already adding up future profits. And lining up future girlfriends.

"Okay, I'll do it," he said. "But not today. Come back at three o'clock tomorrow. We'll do the interview in my office. Come down to the lower entrance."

"I'll be there," I said with a secret sigh of relief. Then I pulled my purse up over my shoulder, said my good-byes, and left the big glass house as quickly as I could. I didn't want to get a sunburn.

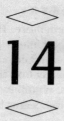

14

I needed a bathroom, a telephone and something to eat, so I drove into downtown Port Washington, to the one restaurant I was familiar with—the coffee shop that used to be the high school hang-out. Expecting the place to be crawling with kids on their lunchbreak, I was surprised to find the counter and most of the booths empty. I went straight to the bathroom in the back and then stopped at the pay phone on my way out, where I punched in the number of the Masterson estate. If Ben answered, I decided, I would just hang up.

Luckily, the maid, Linda, came on the line. I identified myself and asked to speak with Bette Masterson.

"Sorry, Mrs. March, she's not taking any calls today," Linda told me in a hushed, worried voice. "She had a very bad night and we had to call the doctor in first thing this morning. She was in such pain that he gave her a massive sedative. He said she'd be sleeping for the rest of the day."

"I'm very sorry to hear that," I said. "When she does wake up, please tell her that I called to find out how she was."

"I will. She'll be pleased to know you inquired."

"And how about Daisy?" I asked. "Is she at home?"

"No. When the nurse, Dora, saw she wouldn't be needed here for the day, she decided to take Daisy into the city for lunch and a movie. Mr. Ben was also going in, so they went along with him in the limousine. They won't be back until dinnertime."

"Really?" I said, wheels turning in my head. "Oh, mmmmm, gee," I mumbled, stalling for time. Eager to take advantage of the unexpected godsend, I struggled to think up a believable reason for asking to visit the Masterson greenhouse while everybody was gone. Finally, I settled for *not* so believable, unraveling a complicated, long-winded story about how I was a rabid horticulturist, and how Daisy had promised me a cutting from a very special and rare plant we discovered in the greenhouse the other day, and—since I was in the vicinity right now, visiting my dear old dad in nearby Port Washington—would it be too much trouble if I just drove out to the estate, parked my car way out in the back, and stepped inside the greenhouse for a few minutes? I wouldn't have to bother anybody or go up to the big house at all. I would just clip one itty bitty little branch off that wonderful Greek Euonymus shrub and be on my way.

To my great amazement, she fell for it. "That would be just fine, Mrs. March," she said. "You can come over any time you want to." Linda obviously knew even less about plants than I did. There was nothing rare or special about Euonymus shrubs. Practically every yard in Rockville Centre had one. There were at least six of them nestled around *my* little house, which was the only reason I happened to know the name.

I thanked Linda profusely and told her I would be

there in an hour or so. Then, breathless with success and marveling at my newfound nerve, I hung up the phone, took a seat at the lunch counter and started looking over the menu. It hadn't changed much.

"What can I get ya?" the short chubby white-haired man behind the counter asked. "We got turkey today, and vegetable soup."

I recognized the voice before I made out the face. It was Hoppy, the same man who had worked at the coffee shop when I was a senior in high school, more than a quarter of a century ago. His real name was Homer, but all the kids had called him Hoppy, making fun of the fact that—anxious and overworked as he was—he always bounced around the place like a big bunny.

But he wasn't bouncing anymore. And—since I was the only one at the counter and only two of the booths were occupied—you couldn't say he was overworked, either. "Hi," I said, choosing not to embarrass him with the use of his old nickname. "How's it going?"

"Swell," he said sarcastically. "Life's a beach."

"You're not too busy," I observed. "Don't the high school kids come here anymore?"

"Nope. They stopped comin' about fifteen, twenty years ago when they all started gettin' their own cars. Now they spend the whole damn lunch hour tearin' up and down the street with their windows wide open and their radios blastin' so loud it rattles the blinds. Don't know where they eat, *if* they eat. Some fast food place prob'ly."

"Yeah, probably," I said, looking around at the drab, pictureless walls that had once, for a few hours every day, embraced the hopes, dreams, loves, hates, terror, anguish—all the squirming passions of the savage, immortal young. A wave of nostalgia washed over me. I could almost see myself nuzzling with Mitch Campbell in the corner booth while Mary Lee Lumpkin and Binky Sharp practiced basketball cheers in the crowded aisle and the Beatles sang "Help!" in the background.

"So, what'll ya have?" Hoppy asked again.

I ordered a cheeseburger with extra pickles and a side of onion rings for old time's sake.

Turning into the Masterson estate a half-hour later, I saw that Juan was trimming hedges near the entrance. I thought of stopping to ask him if he had been on the premises the night Jane was killed, but decided to wait and try to catch him on the way out. Then I drove a little faster up the long private roadway, hoping to get inside the greenhouse and complete my mission before Juan returned to his adjoining quarters.

I parked the car in the rear driveway, as close to the greenhouse as possible, and darted across the lawn and inside. Remembering that the police believed Jane had been down on her knees when she was shot, I kept my gaze glued to the slatted redwood runner and the floor of brown gravel beneath it as I walked down the first aisle. Nothing unusual caught my eye. I turned the corner and hurried up the next aisle. Then the next, and the next.

It was on the fifth aisle that I found what I was looking for: a break in the predictable pattern, a change in the perfect structure. I froze in my tracks and stared down at the last section of the runner. It had obviously been recently repaired. It had, in fact, been *replaced*. The last five feet or so of the redwood track were made of redder, newer wood and the slats were spaced about an eighth of an inch further apart than all of the others.

Heart pounding, I stepped off the end of the runner,

lifted the boardwalk slightly and lugged it over to one side. Then I dropped down into a squat and started digging around in the exposed layer of brownish red pebbles underneath, sifting huge fistfuls of the small porous stones through my fingers. The gravel looked new or recently washed. I dug deeper and deeper, straining my eyes for signs of blood, which I knew would be difficult to detect since the pebbles themselves were a ruddy color.

I couldn't see what I was searching for, but I could feel it. A slight, almost imperceptible gumminess seemed to coat the pebbles in the deepest layers, making them somewhat tacky to the touch. I grabbed a handful of the stickiest specimens and shoved them in my pocket. Then I quickly filled in the holes and smoothed the gravel flat again.

I was about to stand up and shove the runner back into place when a glimmer of something white caught my eye. It looked like a splinter, a toothpick-sized shaving of wood that might have been chipped from one of the whitewashed walls or window frames. I picked it up and took a closer look. Nausea swelled up in my stomach as I realized what the white splinter was. It was a piece of bone. A piece of *Jane's* bone, I thought, and I almost fainted at the sight of it.

A surly male voice startled me to my senses. "What you doing in here?" Juan demanded, staring at me with wild dark eyes. He was standing at the opposite end of the aisle, with a pair of hedge clippers in one hand and a wadded-up red plaid shirt in the other. His bare chest and forehead were gleaming with sweat. From my squatting position on the floor, he looked very tall and menacing as he slowly, roughly, wiped himself down with his shirt.

When I stood up, however, he was reduced to his real size, which was about five-foot-five. And instead of looking menacing, he looked frightened, which made me feel a whole lot better. "Mrs. Masterson knows I'm here," I told him, using a forceful voice and casually putting my right hand in my jacket pocket—my hand *and* the little sliver of bone it carried. "In fact she asked me to come out and look over the greenhouse," I added, "to make sure Jane's plants were doing all right."

"But why you on the floor? Why you move the plank?" He had a shaky voice and a Spanish accent. South American? Puerto Rican? I couldn't tell.

"I dropped my car keys. They fell through the slats and I had to move the plank to find them."

"Oh," he said, setting the hedge clippers down on a small worktable behind him. He shook out his shirt and put it back on. Then, raking his fingers through his thick black hair, he turned and started to walk away.

"Oh, uh, Juan?" I called, stumbling toward him on the crooked wooden runner. "Can I ask you a question?"

He didn't say anything, but he stopped walking. When he turned toward me I thought I saw a look of fear shoot across his face.

"Did you work late last Thursday?" I asked him. "Were you here the night Miss Masterson was murdered?"

"No!" he insisted. "I already told policeman. I wasn't here. I don't know nothing." His small black eyes flitted around in his face like trapped houseflies.

"What time did you go home?"

"Very early. Only six o'clock."

"When you came to work the next morning did you notice anything strange?"

"Many police cars here."

"Besides that, I mean. Did you see anything unusual around the grounds, or here in the greenhouse?"

"No. Everything the same. Nothing different."

I didn't believe him. Another sheet of perspiration had broken out on his face and neck. A few drops trickled down his cheeks and disappeared into his thick black mustache. The question was, what was he in such a great big sweat about—his own guilty involvement or somebody else's? I knew I wasn't going to get the answer to that question from Juan himself—not yet, anyway—so I thanked him for his time and made a speedy retreat to my car.

As soon as I left the Masterson grounds and hit the public road, I pulled over to the side, stopped the car, and fished around in my purse until I found my makeup bag. Dumping my cosmetics into the bottom of my purse, I wiped out the inside of the small zippered clutch with a tissue and propped it open on the seat beside me. Then I carefully removed the sticky pebbles and the bone splinter from my jacket pocket, placed them in the makeup bag and zipped it closed.

I knew the evidence had been contaminated—with fingerprints, jacket fuzz, tissue fibers, maybe even face powder—but it was the best I could do. I put the small bag back in my purse, carefully anchoring it between my wallet and my hairbrush.

But what the heck was I going to do with it now? Stick it in the closet with Jane's Filofax? I pulled away from the curb and back into traffic, puzzling over my new dilemma. What good is having evidence if you can't prove anything with it? There was no way *I* could run the tests needed to determine if the blood and bone were really Jane's. I wouldn't even be able to tell if the sticky stuff on the pebbles actually *was* blood! With my luck, it would turn out to be corn syrup.

There was only one reasonable thing to do, I decided. Hand the evidence over to Eddie.

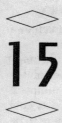

15

I arrived at Nassau County Police Headquarters at about three-thirty. The same two officers were stationed in the security booth near the entrance. I told them who I had come to see and they directed me, once again, to the red-striped phone near the elevators. When I called extension 78, a female voice—the woman with the burgundy hair?—answered. "Homicide," she croaked, sounding like a sea lion with a head cold.

I told her who I was and asked to speak to Detective Sergeant Lincoln. She put me on hold, and a few seconds later, Eddie came on the line.

"Speak of the devil," he said. "Spock and I were just talking about you, wondering if you're ready to confess yet." I could tell from his tone of voice that he was just kidding, so I didn't get upset.

"As a matter of fact I am," I teased. "That's why I'm downstairs in the lobby. Can you spare a few minutes?"

"I'll be right down," he said and hung up.

I was glad he hadn't asked me to come upstairs. I felt

like running into Lieutenant O'Donnell as much as I felt like brushing my teeth with bird droppings.

I walked over to the long wooden bench near the magazine rack and sat down next to the only other occupant—an Elvis lookalike wearing a black leather jumpsuit unbuttoned down to his beltline. He had about sixty gold chains around his neck. I wondered if he was there to be interrogated, to apply for a job, or to entertain the troops.

Within a few moments Eddie appeared at the end of the hall, smiling and walking toward me in his fast and easy gait. My heart started beating in time with his footsteps.

"Come on," he said when he reached my side of the bench. "Let's get out of here." He held out his hand and tucked it under my elbow when I stood up.

"Where are we going?" I asked, allowing him to guide me to the door.

"B.K. Sweeny's," he said, naming a well-known pub-style steakhouse nearby. "I'm going to feed *you* for a change."

The thought of food almost made me gag. The cheeseburger and onion rings I had eaten for lunch were still crouched in my stomach like belligerent outlaws, refusing to clear out of town and move on down the digestive trail. But I didn't tell Eddie I wasn't hungry. The chance to sit across a table from him in a secluded corner of a dimly lit restaurant was too seductive to turn down. I would just order a drink, I decided. I could use a drink. I really *needed* a drink.

Eddie led me out the door, down the steps, around to the rear of the building and over to a gray Taurus parked in the back lot. "We'll take my car," he said. "The unmarked crates are all in use, and restaurant owners get testy if you leave a squad car parked in front of their establishments too long." He opened the passenger door for me and I got in.

The dark blue interior was comfortable and clean. No old newspapers tossed on the back seat, no crumpled-up doughnut bags or Styrofoam coffee cups wedged between the seats, no cigarette butts scattered on the floor. There was something else on the floor, though—a long dangly earring adorned with lots of crystal beads and little silver stars. I picked it up and handed it to Eddie after he slid in behind the wheel.

"Somebody dropped something," I said.

"Oh, thanks," he said. "Claudine's been looking everywhere for that." Eddie cradled the glittering object in the palm of his hand for a few seconds and then gingerly put it in his shirt pocket. This simple act of marital intimacy filled me with loneliness and made my eyes ache. I was—to put it more plainly—so envious I wanted to cry.

"So what did you want to talk to me about?" Eddie asked after we'd been seated in the restaurant for a while. He lifted a frosty mug of draft beer to his mouth and took a deep swallow, keeping his alert brown eyes trained steadily on my face. A hint of a smile tugged at the corners of his lips.

"Well, actually I wanted to give you something," I said.

"A good piece of your mind?"

I laughed. "No, not this time." I took a deep breath and a big gulp of my Bloody Mary. Then I felt around in my purse until my fingers found the zippered edge of my cosmetics case. With what I hoped was an enticing air of intrigue, I pulled the little black bag out of my purse and put it down in the center of the table.

"What's that?" Eddie asked, looking more irritated than intrigued.

"It's important evidence," I said, puffing up with pride. I could hardly wait to see the look of amazement on his face when I told him what I had found and how I had found it. "I believe the contents of this bag will prove that Jane was killed at the Masterson estate, in the greenhouse."

Eddie grinned. "You sound like you're playing a game of Clue: 'I accuse Professor Plum, in the greenhouse, with the lead pipe.'"

"This is no game!" I insisted. "I'm dead serious."

"So what's in the bag?"

"It's a handful of bloody pebbles and a piece of bone," I blurted out, trying to shock him into paying me the proper respect—the same respect he would pay any fellow investigator. "I found it all in one spot, buried in the gravel floor of the Masterson greenhouse, under a redwood runner that had obviously been recently repaired. *Very* recently repaired," I added, hoisting one eyebrow to the hilt. I felt as smart and sassy as Nora Charles, the better half of the droll detective duo in *The Thin Man*.

At that precise moment a waiter appeared at our table, carrying a tray full of food and totally destroying my bid for attention, not to mention my dramatic flair. He put a platter of steak and home fries down in front of Eddie and placed another Bloody Mary in front of me. As he plunked down the ketchup, the Worcestershire, and the steak sauce, I had to move my cosmetics bag to the side of the table, out of the way.

"Are you sure you don't want something to eat?" Eddie asked. "They make a good spinach salad here."

"No, thanks," I said, glowering until the waiter walked away.

When Eddie picked up his knife and fork and cut into his steak without even *mentioning* my bag of evidence (or my remarkable bravery and outstanding powers of deduction), I wanted to reach over and pull his hair. How could he be so indifferent? Didn't he care about catching the murderer anymore? And what the hell had happened to the sensitive guy who was so frantically concerned about my safety? Didn't he realize I had risked my life getting that bloody stuff out of the greenhouse? (Well, I *sort* of had. Ben *could* have come home, and found me in the greenhouse, and pulled out his gun, and so forth, and so on . . .)

My mind was racing with such thoughts, but I didn't put any of them into words. I didn't pull Eddie's hair, either. Remembering what had happened the last time I'd lost my cool with him, when I'd almost incriminated myself by revealing my knowledge of the rape, I decided to sit still and practice a strict vow of silence. I blinked my aching eyes, took a long look around the dark, nearly deserted restaurant, and—except for stealing a few sips of my Bloody Mary—kept my mouth carefully closed.

After what seemed like an hour, but was probably just thirty seconds, Eddie picked up the conversation again. "When did you dig this evidence up?" he asked between mouthfuls of home fries. "This afternoon?"

"Yes."

"Did anybody see you?"

"No, not really. Juan, the gardener, came into the greenhouse and found me scrunched down on the floor, but he didn't know what I was doing. I told him I dropped my car keys."

Eddie suddenly lost interest in his food. He put his fork down on his plate and rubbed his wonderful face with both hands. "Oh God, Annie," he said softly. "Why couldn't you stay out of this? I begged you not to get involved."

I almost got angry, but I didn't. Something in Eddie's voice made me feel nervous instead. And when I spoke, my own voice came out in a raspy whisper. "I didn't *choose* to get involved, you know. Somebody put a dead body in my trunk, and I've been trying to prove my own innocence ever since."

"But you don't have to do that, Annie. That's *my* job."

"Yes, but I feel the need to pitch in. With my link to the Masterson family, I may be in a position to uncover some things that you can't."

"Like the blood and bone samples in that bag?"

"Well, yeah, maybe—"

"We found similar samples five days ago," he said sternly. "They were dug up from the greenhouse floor, in the fifth aisle over from the door, under a section of the wooden walkway that had clearly just been rebuilt. Several bone fragments were found, as well as a few chunks of flesh and gristle, and hundreds of bloody rocks were collected. The whole gory mess has been under microscopic inspection at the Medical Examiner's office since Saturday, and all tests have proved that the flesh, blood, and bone came from the body of one Jane Camille Masterson, deceased."

He paused for a moment, staring at me with intense concentration. Then he leaned forward and drove his point home: "Do you still think you're in a better position to discover the truth than the Nassau County Homicide Squad?"

If I had been standing on the edge of the Grand Canyon at that moment, I might have jumped in. As it was, my pulse started throbbing, my face got hot and I stared down at my paper placemat in shame. Instead of Nora Charles, I felt like Lucy Ricardo.

"And make no mistake about it, Annie, there are a lot of *other* things we already know about this case," Eddie went on. "Things I'm not at liberty to discuss with you. I will tell you, however, that we already know for certain what kind of gun was used. So don't bother going back to the greenhouse to look for the bullet. We found it five days ago when we dug up and sifted through all the other evidence at the crime scene.

"And don't bother hanging around the estate to question Bette Masterson and her sister, Daisy, any-more. We've got them covered. And you can forget about scheduling any more meetings with Ben Masterson at the Garden City Hotel—unless, of course, you just want to go to bed with him." Did I detect a lit-tle note of jealousy in his sarcastic tone? "We've interro-gated Ben thoroughly, investigated his past, and he's still under surveillance twenty-four hours a day," Eddie declared.

"So, you can see we *are* working around the clock on this case," he added, speaking a little more softly. "And we *have* gotten a lot accomplished. And we *will* con-tinue to turn up new evidence and follow every lead until Jane Masterson's murder is solved. I don't mean to hurt your feelings, Annie, but we really don't need your help on this. You're just gumming up the works and putting yourself in danger. Why don't you stick to teaching reading and let *us* handle this investigation?"

"Sounds like I've been under surveillance myself," I said meekly.

"Right."

"But how did you know that other thing?" I asked.

"What other thing?" he asked me back.

"That I'm a reading tutor."

"We talked to the ladies who work in the Hempstead Library on Thursday evenings. Most of them recognized your picture. They said you're a literacy volunteer, and that you've been tutoring a blond black woman there every Thursday evening for the past three or four years. They also told us," he said with a chuckle, "that you and your student get a little unruly sometimes. That if you can't learn to control yourselves, they might have to ask you to look for a new place to study."

My face got a little warmer and, I'm sure, redder. It was just my day, I figured. My day for total embarrassment. "What do you mean, they recognized my picture?" I asked. "What picture?"

"One of the lovely close-ups taken by our still photographer the night you found the body. He snapped a few shots while we were standing and talking in the parking lot. Remember?"

"I wasn't aware that he was taking pictures of *me*."

"There's a lot you aren't aware of," he said, slicing into his steak again.

We sat in silence for a few minutes while Eddie finished eating and I tried to coax my self-esteem into making a comeback. The fact that Eddie kept looking at me and smiling (affectionately, not derisively) helped a lot. I wondered how, as chastened and humiliated as I was, I could still find my tormentor so damn attractive.

"So what should I do with this?" I asked, picking up my cosmetics case and dangling it in the air liked the bag of chicken feed it had become.

"Throw it away."

"You don't want to take it to the Medical Examiner or add it to the other body of evidence?"

"No. It wouldn't help the investigation at all, and it would only cause you more problems."

"Why?" I asked, reactivating my total nitwit status. After everything that had just gone down, after all the painful lessons I had just learned, I still didn't have a clue.

"Think about it, Annie," he said impatiently. "The evidence in that little bag of yours does nothing to further our investigation—nothing but implicate *you*. Don't you see? You knew exactly where to dig the stuff up, and now it's probably got your fingerprints all over it. What do you think the other guys in the department would make of that? Do you really want me to take it back to Headquarters and open up *that* can of worms?

"No, I—"

"Do yourself a favor," he went on. "Chuck that bag and everything in it into the first dumpster you can find."

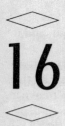

16

A dumpster was out of the question. The tiny traces of blood and bone contained in my cosmetics case had once been a part of Jane's body, for God's sake. I couldn't just throw the bag away. I would bury it in my backyard, I decided, near the spot where Sam and I had buried our first cat, Popeye, when he'd been run over by a UPS truck. I stopped at a nursery on the way home and bought a package of bulbs—dark blue irises—which I planted, along with the bag, as soon as I got back to the house.

Then, still feeling bewildered and embarrassed, I went inside and made myself another Bloody Mary. I sat down at the kitchen table, flipped on the news, and stared at the TV like a zombie while I drank.

I mulled over all the things Eddie had said to me in the restaurant, and I wondered if he was right. Was all my secret snooping just messing up the case instead of helping it? I didn't think so. What harm could have been caused by my little visits with Bette and Daisy? And my two encounters with Ben hadn't done any damage that I could see—except to my modest composure and his groin-centered ego.

Okay, so maybe I hadn't turned up any useful information yet, but that didn't mean I never would. Maybe I'd find out something really important tomorrow, or the next day. Besides, I had a magazine interview to conduct and a feature article to write. Eddie couldn't expect me to stop pursuing my career! Actually, he hadn't mentioned Niles or Nina Stanwyck even once while he was reading me the riot act, so I reckoned I could talk to them, at least, without stepping on Homicide's overly sensitive toes.

I finished my drink, fed the kitties, turned off the television, and lugged my very tired, slightly drunk body into the bedroom. I hadn't had any dinner and it wasn't even seven o'clock, but I decided to get a jump-start on the long night ahead. I flopped down on the bed, curled myself up like a fetus, and fell into a deep black sleep with all my clothes and my cowboy boots still on.

When my doorbell rang at eight forty-five the next morning, yanking me up from a murky sea of dreams, I could barely open my eyes. Somebody had snuck into my bedroom in the middle of the night and spackled my lids together with putty. And filled my head up with sand. And stuffed a lot of feathers in my mouth.

With a great deal of effort, I rolled over to the edge of the bed and forced myself to stand up. I didn't have any idea who was at the door. And as I hobbled into the living room to answer it, I felt—and no doubt looked— like an addled ostrich with boots on.

I cracked open the front door and peeped out. Two young men wearing jeans, sweatshirts, and big leather tool belts were standing on the porch, bristling with purpose and obviously expecting to be admitted to my house.

"Can I help you?" I asked. My words came out in a mumbled mess.

"We're from Safe and Sound," the larger man said. "You wanted an alarm system put in?"

"Oh yeah," I said, pulling the door all the way open. "I forgot you were coming today."

"That's okay," he answered. "So long as you don't forget to pay us." He shot a glance at his skinny dark-haired cohort and they both cracked up laughing. Then they clomped into the house, introduced themselves as Freddy and Raymond, determined what kind of alarm I wanted and got to work on the wiring.

A few minutes later the locksmith arrived with the deadbolts I ordered. His name was Myron. I introduced him to Freddy and Raymond and then he started drilling holes in all the doors. I went into the kitchen, made a pot of coffee for everybody and then locked myself in the bathroom while I washed up. I was still dressed from the day before, so I didn't have to worry about what clothes to put on.

The rest of the morning was a dizzy headache of banging hammers, buzzing drills, and wailing sirens. My little house was trampled, pounded, skewered, and showered with sawdust. And by the time the three men finished their work and left, my brain was dead and my nerve endings were tied in knots. I was four and a half hours older and $1,850 poorer.

But I was protected. Oh, how I was protected! My jumbo ring of house keys was impressive enough to make any jailer jealous. To break in through one of my doors, an intruder would have to either saw or shoot the locks off first. And if anybody ever *did* get one of the doors or windows of my house open, the siren in my attic would howl loud enough to deafen everybody in the tristate area. Minutes later, six carloads of cops would screech to the scene.

I had to laugh at the irony of it all. Unidentified burglars, rapists, and murderers were roaming all over the place, living in complete freedom, while *I* was living in a high security prison.

A bowl of oatmeal and a hot bath helped me return to normal. I wanted to clean the house—vacuum the blanket of sawdust and pulverized plaster from my floors and furniture—but I didn't have time. I also wanted to get dolled up for my interview with Niles Stanwyck—I thought a sexy outfit and glamorous makeup might make him more responsive—but I didn't have time for that either. I pulled on a clean pair of jeans and a pink cotton sweater and struck out for Sands Point again.

When I arrived at the Stanwyck house I parked near the flight of stone-paved steps leading to the lower level. It was exactly three o'clock. I hoped Niles would be there at the office to greet me. I had no desire to renew my acquaintance with the watchdog maid.

I was about to ring the buzzer on the lower level when the door flew open and Niles Stanwyck's boyish face popped out of the shadows. "Good afternoon, Mrs. March," he said. "You're very punctual, aren't you?"

"Yes, I am," I said, "and please call me Annie."

"Oh, well, all right, Annie," he replied, frowning slightly and motioning me inside. "And you can call me Niles, I guess." He was obviously reluctant to relate to me on a first-name basis, but I didn't care. I really didn't feel like bowing to his doctorhood all day. In my book, plastic surgeon is not synonymous with saint.

Niles led the way through a small waiting room into a large office with thick gray carpeting, a black marble-topped desk, and several chrome and leather side chairs. In one corner of the room a plush pink sectional sofa curved languidly around a circular black marble coffee table. The walls were decorated with beveled mirrors and stylish pastel portraits of beautiful women, and all the windows were hung with thick, pale pink drapes which were tightly closed. The entire room was bathed in soft pink indirect lighting.

"You can sit anywhere you please," Niles said, coming to a stop in front of his desk. "The couch is very comfortable." He was wearing a dove-gray three-piece suit with an ice blue shirt and a bright blue tie, the color of which matched his eyes perfectly. I wondered how long he had shopped to find it.

"Thanks," I said, studiously avoiding the sofa and sitting down in a chair near the desk. Comfortable though it may have been, I didn't relish the idea of lounging on the good doctor's love divan.

"I've never done a magazine interview before," Niles said, taking his own seat in the black leather throne behind the desk. "I'm sure it will be quite intriguing, but how does one begin?" He sounded so pompous I wanted to laugh.

"There's really nothing to it," I said, setting my tape recorder on the desk and turning it on. "I'll ask the questions, and you answer them. Feel free to digress at any point or elaborate on anything you wish."

"Yes, all right." Niles sat up taller in his chair, straightened his collar and pushed his charcoal wire-framed glasses higher on his well-formed and perhaps surgically sculpted nose. A golden tan illuminated his youthful face; his cheeks were dented with deep dim-

ples. His platinum gray hair looked as if it had been sil-
vered and permed and his nails appeared to have been
professionally trimmed and glossed. If he hadn't been
so prissy, he might have been attractive.

"First, I think we should get some biographical information," I began. "Your age, education, experience, and
so forth."

"Right," he mused, propping his elbows on the desk
and intertwining the fingers of both hands. "I'm forty-
one years old. I graduated from City College and went
to med school upstate, at the State University of New
York Medical Center. I trained in Facial Plastic and
Reconstructive Surgery at the Montefiore Medical
Center and I was an attending surgeon there until I
opened my own practice six years ago. I now own and
operate the Rebirth Center of Corrective Surgery in
New York City, which employs two other surgeons
besides myself, and I offer additional private checkups
and consultations here, in my home office."

"Are you board-certified? Do you belong to any special associations or societies? Our readers always like to
know that kind of stuff."

"Yes, I have a specialty board certification from the
American Board of Cosmetic Surgery, and I'm a member of the Northeastern Society of Plastic and
Reconstructive Surgeons. I also belong to the American
Society of Liposuction Surgery, and . . . wait a second,"
he said, opening his desk drawer and taking out a thick,
slick magazine-sized brochure. "Here's our promotional
booklet, *The Rebirth Experience*. It has a complete bio
on me, with a list of all my degrees, honors, and mem-
berships. Take a copy home with you. It'll tell you
everything you need to know." He leaned across the
desk and handed me the booklet.

I quickly flipped through its glossy pages. There were close-ups of beautiful young women on every spread and numerous shots of perfectly formed body parts—hips, legs, thighs, breasts, and buttocks. The accompanying copy intimated that all of the faces and bodies in the brochure had been reconstructed at the Rebirth Center but, since none of the photos had captions or identifications of any kind, I recognized the presentation for what it was: a cunning commercial full of bold-faced lies. I would have bet a year's earnings that none of the young models pictured in that booklet had ever been within ten miles of Dr. Stanwyck's scalpel.

That's not to say I thought Niles was a lousy surgeon. Quite the opposite, as a matter of fact. If Jane and Nina offered true examples of his surgical skills and expertise, the man was one smooth operator.

"This article is about body surgery, not facial surgery," I said. "So—ignoring all operations from the neck up—how many different cosmetic reconstructive procedures do you offer, and which are the most popular?"

"There are over a dozen major procedures," Niles said, "and I'm skilled at all of them. Buttock, arm, and thigh lifts; buttock, calf, and pectoral implants; tummy tucks, liposuction, and scar revision; skin transplantation and collagen insertion. There are four different procedures for the breast: augmentation, lift, reduction, and reconstruction.

"And then," he added, "for that special man in your life, there's a wonderful new procedure to extend the length of the penis." Niles suddenly dropped his pretentious decorum and leered openly at me. He looked like a demented goat.

I was surprised by his coarse behavior, but I ignored it and went on with the interview. "Of all the operations you mentioned," I continued, "which types are most frequently requested by your patients?"

He grew pompous again. "Liposuction and breast augmentation are by far the most popular choices," he said. "Not just among my patients, but among women all over the country. They go for liposuction of the thighs, hips, and abdomen and, despite all the bad press about leaking silicone, they still go for breast implants. Over 200,000 women received breast implants in the last year. It's a $600 million a year business."

"I don't believe it," I said. I was truly shocked that so many women would brave the possibility of disease— and even death—just to have bigger boobs.

"Well, it's true," he said. "Just look at all the celebrities who've had breast augmentation surgery—Morgan Fairchild, Mariel Hemingway, Jane Fonda, Brigitte Nielsen, Jessica Hahn, Mary Tyler Moore, Melanie Griffith." He rattled off the names like a teacher taking attendance.

"Knife styles of the rich and famous," I said.

He gave me a wan smile. "You can joke all you want," he replied, "but for some women the size of their breasts is a very serious matter. They know how important beautiful breasts are to most men, and they're willing to do anything to make themselves attractive to their husbands or lovers. I applaud that goal and I'm happy to be able to help so many women achieve it.

"You should see how grateful they are afterward," he added, staring dreamily into the middle of the room and licking his lips repeatedly.

I almost barfed. The man's sanctimonious self-importance was sickening, not to mention his randy

drool. I wondered how Jane could ever have gotten
involved with this creep. Had he been her first lover?
Had her self-esteem been so low, and her sexual experience so lacking, that his perverse attentions just swept
her off her feet? And what was Nina's story? Why did
she stay married to such an unfaithful lout?

"Youth and beauty are the most sought-after com-
modities in the world today," Niles went on, "and I'm
proud to be able to bestow those blessings on a chosen
few." He delivered his sermon from the highest cloud
and, as he spoke, his hands fluttered through the air like
flesh-colored birds. He was wearing three diamond
rings on his left hand alone.

"Can you give me some idea of what the various procedures cost?" I asked, trying to shoot him out of the
sky. "What, for instance, would be the price of a tummy
tuck?"

"Anywhere from $5,000 to $12,000," he said,
"depending on the difficulty of the operation."

"And liposuction?"

"From $2,000 to $10,000."

"What about breast implants?"

"$3,500 to $7,000."

"Sounds pretty steep."

"Yes, but how does one place a value on beauty and
self-image? Besides," he added, "we offer monthly
financing with no money down, a thirty-six-month pay-
back period and 17 percent interest. The interest varies
monthly."

I smiled. Having cosmetic surgery, it seemed, was
sort of like buying a new car. Both undertakings were
expensive, both could take a very long time to pay off,
and both could, under extreme circumstances, lead to
bodily injury and even death.

"But all of this information is in the booklet I gave you," Niles said impatiently. "We really don't have to discuss it." He was getting annoyed at me. I wasn't showing the proper reverence for his talent—or his wealth.

"Then let's move on to the operations themselves," I said. "Can you give me a detailed description of exactly what happens when you're performing a buttocks lift?" *Performing* a buttocks lift. I liked that. "Where do you make the incisions and how, exactly, are the buttocks lifted?"

"We don't have to talk about that, either," he said, scowling. "Every procedure is outlined, in detail, in the booklet. You will have no trouble finding all the information you need for your article. Assuming, that is, that you know how to *read*."

Boy, was he getting testy! I realized I'd have to adopt a more conciliatory tone and start massaging his ego if I wanted to keep the conversation going.

"Are you sure this is your first magazine interview?" I asked him.

"Quite sure," he grunted.

"Then you must have been on TV a lot."

"No, never. But what made you think so?" He straightened his tie and craned his neck in my direction.

"Well, I just can't believe that a man of your immense talent has been so overlooked by the media. Judging from the wonderful work you did on Jane Masterson, and the stunning improvements you made in your own wife's beauty (I was just fishing there, of course), you must be one of the top plastic surgeons in the country, if not the world." For a moment I thought I may have heaped it on too thick, but one look at his face told me he was eating it up, and licking the spoon afterward.

"Jane Masterson was my masterpiece," he said eagerly. "You can't imagine what she looked like when she first came to me."

"I don't *have* to imagine what she looked like," I lied. "I remember when she was a dumpy brunette with a hideous nose. As far as I'm concerned, you're a miracle-worker."

He relaxed into the back of his chair and stretched his mouth into a gummy smile. "She came out perfect, didn't she? Of course she had good bone structure to begin with—that's what made it all possible. But even *I* was surprised that the ugly duckling could be transformed into such a swan. Jane Masterson was my greatest creation."

"What about Nina? She's pretty incredible-looking, too."

"Yes, but she still has some flaws. After her last two operations, Nina developed quite a bit of scarring on her stomach and thighs. Jane's young flesh healed so quickly and evenly that her scars became virtually imperceptible. Also, Nina is too short. There was nothing *I* could do about *that*. Jane, on the other hand, was the perfect height—tall enough to look regal and graceful without towering over the average man."

"Her death must have come as a terrible shock to you."

"You'll never, never know how I've suffered," he said in a near-whisper. "Mere words can't express how much she meant to me. I'll never find another patient like Jane. I just can't believe she's gone. All that work for nothing . . ." He was pouting like a little boy who'd lost his favorite toy.

"Do you have any idea who killed her?"

"No," he said, tossing nervous glances around the

room. "None whatsoever." He raised his right hand to his mouth and started chewing on the cuticle of his manicured thumbnail.

"Do you know *why* anybody would want to kill her?"

"No."

"Do you think Ben had anything to do with it?"

"I don't know what you're talking about."

"Did Jane ever say anything—"

"Look," he broke in, "I really don't want to talk about it, okay? I'm trying to get over it now. I want to forget about what happened, not study it from every possible angle. Let's get back to the magazine interview. Do you have any more questions about surgical procedures?"

"Well, no, I—"

"Did you ever think of having surgery yourself?" he interrupted again.

"No! I really don't like the idea of—"

"That's too bad," he said. "An eye lift would do wonders for your expression. And your jawline could use a little refinement. I also noticed, when you first walked in, that your behind is starting to sag a bit."

His cutting remarks had the effect he was probably aiming for. Cringing with aversion—and acute self-consciousness—I gathered my stuff together, thanked him for his time, and left without mentioning the murder again.

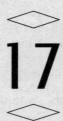

17

The drive home was a pleasure. I whizzed along the Expressway like a woman with the world on a string. As far as I was concerned, my afternoon mission had been a crackerjack success. I had all the facts, figures, and quotes I would need to write a cover story for Ellen, plus I had a fairly clear understanding of what the relationship between Niles and Jane had really been like.

Their affair had been intense, I figured, but not very tender or romantic. She had loved him in the way a Muslim loves Mohammed, and he had loved her in the way a composer loves his latest symphony. I was certain that Niles knew or at least suspected something about Jane's murder, but I didn't think he had taken part in it. He was far too proud of his "masterpiece" to have willfully destroyed her.

It was a balmy late afternoon and rush hour hadn't really started cooking yet. The Meadowbrook Parkway was as clear as a takeoff runway. Flashing a grateful smile at the newly green trees and the peach-colored sky, I pushed a Joe Cocker cassette in the tape deck and sang my lungs out all the way home. Life was a breeze.

Getting into my house, on the other hand, turned out to be a little tricky. First I had to unlock the regular door lock. Then I had to unlock the deadbolt lock. And then, in order to disarm the alarm and keep the siren from going off, I had to punch my secret four-digit code into the number pad mounted near the front door. The problem was that my secret code had somehow, during the course of the day, become a total secret to me.

I madly poked a bunch of random numbers into the system, hoping intuition would guide my finger to hit the right sequence. No such luck. The siren went off right on schedule—exploding my eardrums, ripping the neighborhood peace to shreds, and scaring my cats right out of their skins. Tails frizzed and paws scrambling, they zipped into my bedroom and scooted under the bed. I wanted to do the same thing, but I was frozen in place with my fingers in my ears.

By some miracle, I still managed to hear the telephone ring. Leaving the front door standing wide open, I dashed into the kitchen to answer it. It was the central station watchman at the alarm company. He knew my alarm had been triggered and he demanded to know my secret code *word*, or he would notify the police of a break-in. I remembered that much, at least. "Dixie," I said, and thanked the fellow for his vigilance. Then I rummaged through my catch-all kitchen drawer until I found the slip of paper I had written the secret *number* down on.

Hurtling back toward the front door to turn off the siren, I plowed into a strange hulking thing standing right in the middle of the living room. It was a man. A very big man. A very big, ugly man with a long, narrow head, bulldog jowls, and biceps the size of buffaloes. He was holding a gun in one of his huge meaty hands. When he grabbed me by the arm with his other hand, I screamed my head off.

I cried out as loud as I could, but the alarm screamed louder, reducing my cries to whimpers. I struggled to get away from the man, but it was hopeless. Baring his crooked yellow teeth in a hideous smile, he held on to me as easily as a bear trap holds on to a rabbit. That's when the full horror of my predicament blasted into my brain. I was in the grips of a psychotic madman—Ben's hit man, I believed—and, thanks to my alarm company's watchful efficiency, the police would *not* be zooming to my assistance.

No words could describe my terror. I looked up into my attacker's feral face and relived my whole life in an instant. I even caught a glimpse into the near future, when I would be raped, murdered, and laid to rest in Nassau Knolls Cemetery, right next to Jane. The blood drained out of my head, my knees turned into pulp and I passed out.

When I came to, I was lying flat on my back on one of the couches in my living room. The alarm wasn't shrieking anymore. The front door was closed and Katy Kat was sitting on the arm of the couch staring down at me. Surprised to be alive, and relieved to discover that I still had all my clothes on, I stayed immobile for a few seconds, straining my ears for sounds of the rapist–hit man. All I could hear was the drone of the oil burner. I sat up too quickly and went blind, my vision crackling with little stars.

"Feeling better?" a deep male voice boomed from the direction of the kitchen. I flinched and almost fainted again.

"Sorry I scared you so much," the voice said, moving closer. "But I'm under orders to take special care of you, see? So when your alarm went off and I found your front door wide open, I had to come in and check out the scene."

My eyes returned to normal and I saw that the big ugly man was standing right in front of me, holding one of my Mickey Mouse mugs in his giant paw.

"I made you some hot tea," he said, setting the cup down on the coffee table. "Drink up. It'll do you good."

Hot tea? Ben's hit man made me hot tea? My mind still wasn't functioning too well. It took me a few more seconds to grasp the fact that the man was probably friend, not foe.

"Who are you?" I asked. My voice was raspy from screaming so hard.

"Name's Hobbs. Detective Lou Hobbs."

"You're with the police?"

"Sure am. Been with the NCPD over thirty years. Used to be in Narcotics, but I'm in Homicide now."

"Oh," I said. "You work with Eddie."

"Right. Link—I mean Sergeant Lincoln—is my boss. He's the one told me to take good care of you. Said if anything happened to you he'd demote me to meter maid. 'Course, he didn't mean that. That's just Link's way of keeping me on my toes."

I smiled. It was nice to know Eddie was looking after me, even if his designated bodyguard *had* almost given me a heart attack. I took a sip of tea, leaned back against the couch cushions and melted with relief. "How did you turn the alarm off?" I asked.

"Used the code number on the piece of paper I found in your hand," he said, pulling a cigarette out of the pack in his shirt pocket and sticking it in the corner of his large rubbery mouth. "You should'a picked your birthday or something. That way you would'a remembered it." Lighting his cigarette with a beat-up old Zippo, he inhaled deeply, exhaled loudly, and widened his wobbly jowls in a grin. His teeth were the color of corn.

"How long was I unconscious?"

"Just a couple'a minutes. Nothin' to worry about. You're hunky-dory now." He took another drag on his cigarette, walked over to the front door and opened it. "Guess I'll be gettin' back to the car. They might be tryin' to reach me on the radio."

"Oh, well, uh . . . thanks for the tea, Detective Hobbs."

"Sure thing, Toots. Take care of yourself, and learn that alarm code." He stepped out on the porch and closed the door behind him. I watched him through the blinds as he lumbered down the driveway and folded his hulking body into the dark blue Chevy sitting at the curb.

Later that evening I went to meet Philly at the library. "Let's get out of here," I said to her as soon as I found her hunched over a book at a corner table. "I haven't had a thing to eat since one-thirty this afternoon. Let's go have our lesson at the diner."

"That's fine with me, babe." She slapped her book closed and stood up. After pulling on a turquoise windbreaker over her uniform, she stuffed her books and papers into a big orange tote bag. "I'm kinda hungry myself," she said, talking over her shoulder as she led the way to the library exit. "I'm gonna get me some pancakes."

It wasn't completely dark yet, but you could already

see the stars. And the sideways smile of the moon. As Philly and I walked through the library parking lot near the area where we had discovered the body, we didn't say a word. The all-too-vivid memory of Jane's bloody chest, shattered spine, and empty eyes stunned us both into silence. Could it really have been only one short week ago that we found her? It seemed more like a century.

We took both cars to a diner on Hempstead Turnpike and reconvened inside, in a booth at the back of the restaurant.

"The roast pork sandwich sounds good," Philly said, pouring over the menu, "but I'm still gonna get me some pancakes." She raised her head and gave me a funny look. "Would you believe I used to order a hamburger every time I went out to eat? I couldn't read the dang menu, and I didn't want to make a fool of myself by askin' somebody to read it to me. But I'm makin' up for lost time now," she said, beaming. "I haven't had a nasty old hamburger in two years."

A skinny waitress with gray steel wool hair suddenly materialized at our table. She wore a scowl on her face and a name tag on her chest that said Lola. "Whaddaya want?" she demanded, taking an order pad out of her apron pocket. "We're all out of corned beef hash," she said with a smirk, as if hoping that bit of news would send us running from the restaurant in tears.

Showing no reaction to the corned beef hash deficit, Philly ordered pancakes and I ordered a chef's salad. With obvious disappointment, the wiry old waitress marched off toward the kitchen.

"Let's get started on our lesson," I said as soon as she was gone. "I wish we could pick up where we left off last week, but all the workbooks and flash cards were in my car when it was impounded by the police. We'll have to improvise."

I unzipped my purse and started looking around for the note Philly had left me after she spent the night. I found it flattened against the side of my bag, right next to the map I had used to get to the Stanwycks' house. I took both the note and the map out of my purse and put them on the table.

First we worked on the note, reading it over out loud together. I gave Philly the correct spellings of *tomorow* and *sootcase*, and she practiced writing both words on a paper napkin. Then we began studying the map: how to tell north from south; how to use the color chart and the position grid; how to gauge the miles, etc. The little local map was a perfect study aid. It wasn't overwhelming in size or in the amount of data presented, and the names of streets, parks, and waterways were printed in large, easy-to-read typefaces. I was showing Philly how I had used the map to find the Stanwyck house when Lola trudged over to our table and plunked our plates down in front of us.

"You want some dressing for that salad?" she asked me. "We got everything but Blue Cheese. We're all out of Blue Cheese." She eagerly watched my face for signs of a letdown.

"I hate Blue Cheese dressing," I said just to bug her. "I'll have vinaigrette."

"Hummpf," she muttered, plodding toward the kitchen again.

"Ain't she somethin'?" Philly said, squirting syrup all over her pancakes. "If she got any meaner, they'd have to make her a supervisor at the Hempstead nursin' home."

◦   ◦   ◦

After eating, we ordered some coffee and went back to our map lesson. Remembering from my tutor training sessions that maps are especially hard to read since most of the terms used are *names* rather than recognizable words, I tried to focus our study on streets which were named after things instead of people: Oak Tree Lane, Beach Road, Cow Neck Road, etc. The street the Stanwycks lived on—Half Moon Lane—fit this formula, and Philly read the words easily.

Two cups of coffee each and forty-five minutes later, we decided to wrap it up and head for home. I gave Philly the map to take with her, plus two homework assignments involving route planning and following directions.

"You're comin' home with me, aren't you, babe?" she asked when we got out to the parking lot. "Woodrow said you can stay with us long as you want to. We don't have a guest room, but the couch in the livin' room opens up to a bed, and Woodrow's daughter, Jewel, says it's comfy as a old sneaker. And I know she's tellin' the truth 'cause she stays with us a week every Christmas and she sleeps like a drunk baby."

"It's great of you and Woodrow to invite me," I told her, "and I really do appreciate the offer, but there's no reason for me to leave my house now. I had deadbolt locks and a burglar alarm installed this morning. My house is a freaking fortress. I'll be safer there than anywhere," I said, wondering if that was true. The incident with Detective Hobbs hadn't exactly bolstered my faith in alarm systems.

"Are you sure, girl? I'd still feel better if you came home with me. Won't you get scared bein' in the house all by your own self? We don't have any alarms, but I got a loud voice and Woodrow's got a big baseball bat."

I laughed. The idea of having company did sound pretty nice. But I had cats to feed. And a feature article to write. And a telephone to answer. The hope that Eddie would call or come over seemed to have claimed a permanent place in my psyche.

"I'm sure I'll be fine," I said. "But if I get too scared to stay by myself, you'll be the first to know. Don't be surprised if I show up on your doorstep in the middle of the night with my Rolling Stones T-shirt on."

"Bring a six-pack with you, babe."

I managed to get into my house without setting off the alarm, but I didn't get to the phone in time. I heard it ringing from the front porch, but when I finally got the locks open, punched in the secret code number, and raced to answer it, the line was dead. My new security system had not only caused my near death by heart failure, I decided, but it had also robbed me of the pleasure and excitement of a phone call from Eddie—thereby causing a different kind of heart failure.

I was hanging up my jacket and cursing the crazy, unsafe ways of the world that had forced me to get an alarm in the first place, when the phone rang again. The welcome sound set off some warm emotional reflexes and made my hormones happy. Certain it was Eddie, I dashed into my bedroom, grabbed the portable phone off the night table, and flopped down full-length on the bed. Breathlessly pushing the respond button and holding the handset to my ear, I answered in the softest, sexiest voice I could muster without *totally* embarrassing myself.

"Hellohhhhh?"

"Hi, sweetheart," Ben said. "Did I wake you up? You sound sleepy."

"No!" I cried, jumping to my feet. "I'm not sleepy. And I'm not your sweetheart, either! Why are you calling me? What the hell do you want?"

"Cool down, Dixie. I'm just calling to apologize."

"What?"

"I'm calling to apologize," he repeated. "I'm really sorry for the way I acted the other night. I was out of bounds."

"Out of bounds? You call attempted rape *out of bounds*? What do you call it when you actually commit the rape, *a touchdown*?"

He chuckled. "Always quick with a comeback, aren't you?"

"I wasn't aiming for a comeback," I told him. "And I certainly wasn't trying to make you laugh. I was just trying to point out how despicable your behavior was."

"I know it was, Annie. And that's why I'm calling. It's not easy for me to apologize like this, but I knew I was a bad boy and I needed to talk to you. I'm really sorry for what I did. Please say you'll forgive me."

I didn't want to forgive him. I wanted to throw the book at him. I wanted to shout his guilt from the rooftops and help the police prosecute him—to the full extent of the law—for the rape and murder of his half sister. But if that was ever going to happen, I realized, I would have to see him again. I would have to root around in his vicinity for more evidence, spend some time with him, talk to him some more. And if *that* was ever going to happen, I would have to forgive him first. Or pretend to, anyway.

"I'll forgive you if you forgive me," I said, trying to sound kind of flirty. The effort turned my stomach.

"Forgive you? What for?"

"You know. For popping you in the peanuts."

He laughed. "I got what I deserved.'"

He deserved worse than that, but I didn't say so. What I said was, "I'm not sorry for protecting myself, but I am sorry if I hurt you."

"Oh, you hurt me, all right! But I got over it. You know what they say: 'You can't keep a good man down.'"

Ugh!

"And you know what else they say," he added. "'You only hurt the ones you love.' So I guess I should be flattered by what you did to me."

No, you should get sick and die.

"So how's about it, Annie?" he went on. "Can we bury the hatchet?"

In your crotch.

"Let's have dinner tomorrow night and let bygones be bygones." The man's supply of trite expressions was limitless.

"I'm busy tomorrow night," I lied.

"Then when can we get together? I really need to see you. I've decided to take that job in London—I'll be moving over there in a couple of weeks—and there's something important I want to talk to you about before I leave."

"I'm free for breakfast. Why don't I come out to your place? Your *servants* could make us some eggs or something." I hoped that didn't sound too sarcastic. "And Bette and Daisy could join us. I'd really like to see them again."

"Forget about it! I don't want the old bags hanging around."

"No bags, no breakfast."

"Hey! What's the deal here? Are you afraid to be alone with me?"

"You could say that."

"Really?"

"Yeah, *really*."

"Huh! Well, I guess that's understandable. I'm very disappointed, but . . . well, okay—if that's the way you want it, that's the way it'll be. Breakfast with Bette and Daisy. Ten o'clock tomorrow morning. I'm not crazy about the idea, but I'll just have to pay the piper," he said, trotting out another battered prize from his cliché collection.

"The best things in life are free," I said just to confuse him.

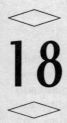

18

Being followed by the police is a disconcerting experience. You feel exposed, reckless, confused, and important—all at the same time. My first reaction when I realized that Spock, or Hobbs—or *somebody* driving the familiar dark blue Chevy—had pulled onto the Expressway behind me was to start planning another pedal-to-the-floor getaway. I didn't want Eddie to find out I was going to the Masterson estate again.

But I soon had second thoughts. Why try to escape? I wasn't doing anything wrong. I was having breakfast with an old school chum and two old ladies. If the police wanted to make a big deal out of that, let them! Spock could stay on my tail all day for all I cared.

Actually, I hoped he would. I'd feel safer that way. What if the real reason Ben wanted to see me this morning was to even the score for what happened in the hotel ladies' room? He could be planning to poison my omelette or drown me in Manhasset Bay. Or gun me down in the greenhouse, for God's sake. But I wouldn't have to worry so much about Ben's hidden agenda if a homicide detective was hovering nearby to protect me.

I checked the rearview mirror several times to make sure that Spock, or Hobbs, or whoever, was still there and—happy to see that he *was*—I drove into the heart of Sands Point with renewed calm and a strong sense of purpose. With Ben moving to London in two weeks, I was going to have to work fast.

Linda greeted me at the door of the Masterson mansion and invited me inside. "They're waiting for you in the breakfast room," she said. I followed her across the entrance hall and into a wide corridor to the right of the stairs. "How did everything go the other day?" she asked as we walked down the dark hall. "Did you get the rare plant cutting you wanted?"

"I sure did. It's now sitting in a glass of water on my windowsill, sprouting roots and soaking up the sun. It'll be a full-grown shrub soon, thanks to you."

"Glad to be of service," she said, smiling. "And I'm also glad you've come to see Mrs. Masterson again. She really needs some human contact, and you're the only one who's visited her since the funeral. Can you believe that?"

"Murder frightens people," I said, remembering how many friends had deserted me after Sam was killed. "They don't know what to say, so they just stop calling."

Coming to a stop outside the last room off the corridor, Linda stood in the open doorway and announced my arrival. I thanked her and went inside.

"Welcome, dear," Bette said from her seat at the huge round table in the center of the sunlit room. "I'm so happy you're here. Come sit next to me."

"No!" Daisy cried, jumping out of her chair and dashing over to grab my hand. "I want her to sit next to me!" She tugged on my arm like a willful child.

Ben stood up from the table, pulled out the chair next to his, and shot me a crooked smile. "*I'm* the one who invited her," he said firmly, "so she's sitting right here, by me." He looked very handsome in his baggy black trousers and purple silk shirt. He also looked determined to have his own way. To save us all from further conflict, I walked over to the chair Ben had pulled out for me and sat down. Daisy reluctantly released my hand and shuffled back to her own place on the other side of the large table.

"Do you want a mimosa?" Ben asked. "I'm having one." To prove his words, he pulled an open bottle of champagne from a silver ice bucket and filled the long-stemmed glass sitting next to his plate. Then he topped it with a little fresh orange juice and took a big gulp.

"I'll just have juice," I said.

"This is quite a treat for me," Bette said, her sad gray eyes flashing a tiny spark of pleasure. "I usually have breakfast alone in my room. It's a very lonely way to start the day. This feels like a party."

"Some party!" Daisy complained. "It's just a stupid old breakfast. We don't have any decorations at all. I bet we don't have any ice cream, either. And how come Dora's not here? Wasn't she invited?"

"No, she wasn't," Ben said. "This party's just for family and old friends." He turned toward me and gave me one of his lascivious winks.

"Dora's an old friend," Daisy grumbled. "She's my *best* friend. I don't see why she can't eat with us."

"Oh, shut up, Daisy!" Ben said. He spit the words out of his mouth as if they tasted bad. "And stop pouting. If you can't behave yourself and have a good time with us, why don't you just leave? Go upstairs and have breakfast with your best friend Dora!"

"All right, I will!" she cried. She slapped her napkin down on the white linen tablecloth, blasted out of her chair, and shoved it back behind her with her legs. "You're so mean," she wailed, pulling at the sleeves of her red Madonna sweatshirt and scrunching her face. "Everything's been awful since you came back home. Only bad things have been happening. I hate you!" Hot tears sprang to her eyes and she ran out of the room before they could spill down her wrinkled cheeks.

Daisy's outburst put a pall over the party. We sat in silence as one of the kitchen maids served the croissants, strawberries, scrambled eggs, and hash browns. Babbling inanely about the good food and beautiful weather, I kept the small talk going while Bette and I ate. Ben chugalugged mimosas and chain-smoked Marlboros.

"Daisy's such a bitch," he said, pouring himself another champagne refill. "Always moaning about something. And always losing her temper, too."

"She can't help it, dear," Bette said. "We must try not to upset her."

"Oh, we *must*, must we?" he mocked. "Well, I'm sick of tiptoeing around her goddamn mental condition! If it was up to me, I'd put the old bat right back in the loony bin."

"Please don't say that, Benjamin!" Bette pleaded. "Daisy's been so happy living here. I love having her with me, and she's no trouble at all, really. No more trouble than any young girl would be. All she needs is someone to keep an eye on her."

Bette's voice quaked with fear as she tried to soften her stepson's anger. Her face twitched and her hands shook uncontrollably. With a flash of insight I saw how completely Jane's death had altered the family power structure. Without the insurance and protection of Jane's love—without Jane's youth, strength, and financial position in the family—Bette and Daisy were at Ben's mercy. And Ben was as merciful as Homer Simpson was smart. If Bette died soon—and probably even if she *didn't*, I realized—Daisy's days of freedom were numbered.

"Have you told Daisy that Dora's leaving?" I asked Bette.

"Oh, my dear, no!" she cried. "I'm afraid of what she'll do. The news will devastate her."

"When is Dora going? Have you found anybody to replace her yet?" I asked.

"She leaves in three weeks and I still haven't hired a replacement. I haven't had any time for interviewing, what with the police and the funeral and all . . ." Bette's watery eyes dissolved into deep pools of pain.

"Well, you'd better find somebody pretty damn fast," Ben growled, "or I'm shipping your crazy sister out of here. She gets on my nerves." He grabbed hold of his glass and downed the rest of his mimosa.

It was right then, at that precise moment—as I sat there watching Ben threaten his stepmother and swill champagne—that the lightbulb lit up over my head. And it wasn't just an ordinary old lightbulb, either. It was one of those super-bright, long-life, compact fluorescent things. A dazzling and brilliant 2000 watt idea.

"I know somebody who'd be good for the job," I said.

"You do?" Bette squeaked, grasping at my words as if they were a lifeline.

"Yes, and I think she'd be happy to work for you."

"Really? Oh, but that's wonderful! Who is she? What's her name, dear?"

"Hang on a second!" Ben bellowed. "Just keep your

fucking pants on. Nobody's getting hired around here unless *I* say so."

He had a lot of nerve telling us to keep our pants on, when *his* were figuratively unzipped and pulled down around his knees at all times. "The decision is yours, of course," I said to pacify him, "but I should think you'd be anxious to hear about *any* prospective candidate since you're moving to London soon. And have you forgotten that Dora is Bette's *nurse* as well as Daisy's companion? Who's going to take care of your stepmother when Dora's gone?"

"There are plenty of nursing agencies around."

"Sure, and they represent lots of bad nurses, too. It's really hard to find a good one, and it's particularly hard to find one who will *stay*. The person I'm thinking of is very loyal and reliable. She's been a nurse's aide at the same nursing home for over fifteen years."

"A nurse's *aide*?" Ben scoffed. "Then she's not a nurse at all. She's not qualified to take care of a cancer patient."

"Dora's not a licensed nurse, either, dear," Bette interjected. Her voice was as thin and crinkly as rice paper. "She wears a uniform, but she's actually just a caretaker—someone to help me clean up and get dressed; someone to comfort me and remind me to take my pills. And that's all I need, really. Whenever I feel sick or have excessive pain, the doctor is always called in."

"See?" I said to Ben. "A licensed nurse is unnecessary. Besides, you'd never find one who'd be willing to care for a physically ill patient and baby-sit a confused old woman at the same time."

I could tell from Ben's face he was starting to cave in. His jaw slackened, his brow relaxed, and his eyes got that glassy look. Chalking his weakening condition up to an entire bottle of champagne, plus my own bubbling powers of persuasion, I went in for the kill.

"Philomena is a wonderful person," I told him. "She's honest, intelligent, diligent, considerate, and fun to be around. Daisy would love her. She's been keeping people clean, comfortable, and happy for fifteen years, and her rates are very reasonable. What more could you ask for?"

"Tell her to call me," Ben yielded, slurring his words and fiddling with his gold hoop earring. "I might give her a whirl."

I had found a possible new nurse for Bette and a new job opportunity for Philly, but I hadn't found any new clues to the crime. Not wanting to go home empty-handed, without a single shred of new evidence to show for my efforts, I excused myself from the breakfast table and dashed upstairs to the bathroom. I figured I'd hide out there for a few seconds and then, taking care to avoid being seen by Dora or Daisy, I'd go looking for Ben's bedroom. As it turned out, however, I didn't have to hide from anybody or go looking for anything. I found all the evidence I could hope for right there in the bathroom.

There was a man's hairbrush sitting on the white tile counter that looked like it hadn't been cleaned in years. I knew it was Ben's because it was matted with long strands of light brown hair. Raking my fingers through the bristles of the brush, I pulled out a handful of hair and carefully wrapped the dandruff-speckled clump in a long strip of toilet paper. I didn't have a cosmetic case anymore, so I stuffed the toilet paper package inside my little green leather coin purse and shoved *that* to the bottom of my shoulder bag. Then I washed my hands and plotted my next move.

I would give the thatch of hair to Eddie, of course, and he would send it out for DNA testing. I had noticed that many of the hairs had their roots intact, and I knew from an article I had written for *Redbook* that this would make for quicker and more conclusive test results. Determining the DNA pattern of the hair might not prove whether or not Ben *killed* Jane, but it would definitely prove—once compared with the DNA pattern of the semen found in Jane's body—whether or not he *raped* her.

I went back downstairs humming the theme music for *Murder, She Wrote*. As I headed down the hall to return to the breakfast room, Ben lunged out of a small dark study on the right, pulled me into the room with him and slammed the door shut behind us.

"Oh, not again, Masterson!" I groaned, trying to sound casual and cocky instead of scared silly, like I really was. "This is getting really boring."

"Oh, yeah?" he said, swaying drunkenly on his feet and grabbing the edge of a tall bookcase for balance. "Well, don't get your hopes up. I'm not gonna attack you again. I just wanna talk to you for a couple'a minutes. Alone." He leaned his face so close to mine I could see all the way up his nose. His breath smelled like rotten fruit.

"Okay, shoot," I said, immediately regretting my choice of words.

"I just wanna tell you I'm gonna miss you . . . when I move to London," he mumbled.

"That's nice," I said, although I really didn't think it was.

"I wantcha ta come over there and visit me next month."

"What?"

"Wantcha ta come visit me."

"Oh, I don't think so, Ben."

"I'll pay for everything."

"It's not the money," I said. "It's just that I'm too busy to travel right now. I've got so many responsibilities . . . you know how it is."

"Yeah! I know how it is," he sputtered. "You don't wanna see me. You don't even wanna know me." He waved his free hand wildly in the air.

He was right, but I wasn't about to admit it. "I don't know what you're talking about," I said.

"I wanna know how come you don't like me," he blubbered. "How come you *never* liked me. I always liked you, y'know. Thought you were the sweetest thing on two feet. Wanted you real bad."

"I liked you just fine," I protested halfheartedly. "I kidded around with you in English class and I laughed at all your jokes."

"Butcha never really *looked* at me," he said. "You hardly even knew I was there."

"You're nuts," I said, growing tired of his game and getting nervous about where it might be heading. I turned away from his rotten breath and moved toward the door.

"Just a minute!" he cried, lurching in my direction. "Where d'ya think you're goin'?"

"To say good-bye to Bette," I answered.

"You're not goin' anywhere," he insisted, trying to grab my arm and stumbling over his own feet in the process. His right hand found my shoulder and held on for dear life. "You can't leave till you gimme a kish."

I didn't have to knee him in the balls to defend myself this time. All I had to do was poke my index finger into the center of his chest and push hard. Arms flailing and legs floundering, he went reeling backwards and crashed into a small antique rolltop desk. Then he slumped like a rag doll to a sitting position on the floor. As I yanked open the door and backed out into the hall, a tiny Tiffany lamp fell off the desk and hit him on the head.

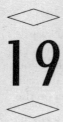

19

As soon as I left the Masterson estate, I drove to the nearest gas station and popped into the public phone booth. After getting the number of police headquarters from information, I shoved a quarter into the rusty slot of the corroded phone and called Eddie. He wasn't there, so I asked to speak to Detective Hobbs.

"Link went to Florida for a couple'a days," Hobbs told me. "Don't know when he'll be back."

My heart sank into my stomach. Eddie must have changed his mind about taking a new job and moving to Ft. Lauderdale. He must have flown down south for a romantic house-hunting weekend with Claudine. I imagined the two of them looking at pink or turquoise ranch houses all morning and lingering on the beach all afternoon. I could picture Claudine's oiled and golden breasts spilling out of her string bikini top, while Eddie's sunblock-coated skin germinated a new crop of freckles.

"Please ask him to call me as soon as he gets back," I said, hoping Hobbs wouldn't notice my whimper.

"Sure thing, Toots."

After returning to my car, I pulled out into the traffic on Port Washington Boulevard, feeling so depressed I almost started crying. I probably would have tortured myself with sunbaked visions of the lovestruck Lincolns all the way home if a white Mercedes hadn't suddenly peeled around me and speeded ahead, giving me a good look at its REBIRTH license plate.

I didn't see who was driving the car, so I decided to follow it for a while and find out. Staying a couple of cars behind the Mercedes (as Spock, or Hobbs, or whoever, had unknowingly taught me to do), I tailed the vehicle across Northern Boulevard, up Searingtown Road and into the rear parking lot of the Americana Shopping Center.

The Mercedes pulled into a parking spot near the back entrance to Barneys and Nina Stanwyck got out. She was wearing an ivory-colored trench coat and a pair of black-rimmed sunglasses. With her collar pushed up and her head held down, she went into the store.

I pulled into a parking spot two lanes behind hers, wondering if Nina was currently under police surveillance. Then I checked behind me to see if *I* was being followed as well. The dark blue Chevy was nowhere in evidence, so I couldn't tell for sure. I smiled at the thought of Nina being tailed by a detective, being tailed by me, being tailed by a detective. A ridiculous convoy, indeed. One nitwit following another.

But I was having fun, I realized. I had stopped fretting about Eddie and Claudine, and my blood was racing with the thrill of the chase. I snatched a tissue out of my purse and wiped off all my lipstick. I pulled my hair back behind my ears and fastened it, with a rubber band, into a short fat ponytail at the nape of my neck.

Then I put on my tortoiseshell-framed eyeglasses and checked myself out in the rearview mirror.

Pretty awful. Looks-wise, I mean. As a disguise, it was pretty good. I considered trying to black out one or two of my front teeth, but decided that would be overkill.

Buttoning my faded gray canvas jacket all the way up under my chin, I got out of the car. Then I tucked my head down between my hunched-up shoulder pads and scuttled—like a sneaky little sand crab—into the store.

The elegantly dressed, perfectly coifed saleswoman stationed near Barneys' back entrance looked me over with an obvious air of aversion. Only the desire to keep her job prevented her from holding her nose.

"May I help you?" she asked, grimacing. Left to follow the true dictates of her heart, she wouldn't even talk to unfashionable people, much less serve them.

"Just looking," I said, grinning. It gave me pleasure to annoy her. If I hadn't been anxious to find Nina I would have stopped long enough to inspect (and unfold) every $200 T-shirt on the display table nearby.

Hurrying past the locked glass jewelry cases and the shelves of absurdly priced accessories, I spotted Nina on the far side of the separates department, going through a rack of sheer black blouses. I moseyed around the shoe section for a while, admiring the butter-soft suede and leather slip-ons, and keeping Nina in sight all the time. After a few minutes of deliberation, she picked out an armload of tops and went into the dressing room.

I didn't think it wise to follow her in there, so while she was gone I went over to check out the items remaining on the rack that had interested her so much.

Some of the blouses were soft and smooth and some were scratchy and pleated. All of them were completely see-through. The cheapest one was priced at $1,248, and—unless you were a prostitute or a porn star—you'd *still* have to buy some other kind of top to wear under it.

As I was gaping at the price tags, Nina swept out of the dressing room and glided up the aisle toward the front entrance of the store. I fell in behind, following her through the men's department and out the door to the front sidewalk. Turning left as she had done, I trailed her down the walk a few yards into Millie's, a restaurant that caters to the tricolor salad and sun-dried tomato crowd.

It was lunchtime, so the restaurant section was packed. The bar, on the other hand, was empty. Nina headed straight for it and took a seat on one of the wooden cane-backed barstools. "I'll have the usual, Rick," she said to the handsome young ponytailed bartender. "But make it a double."

As Rick filled a tumbler-sized glass with Chivas and set it in front of her, I quietly took a seat at the bar, a few stools down from Nina. The wall behind the liquor display featured a mural of a naked woman instead of the usual mirror, so I figured if I kept my head slightly turned and my chin propped in my hand, Nina wouldn't be able to see my face. I ordered a club soda with lime.

A few seconds later a huge man dressed all in black, with a thin dark mustache and a close-shaved head, entered the restaurant and sat down right next to Nina. "Hello, you gorgeous young thing!" he bellowed. I thought he was talking to Nina, but when he added, "The ponytail's to die for!" I realized his remarks were aimed at the bartender. "Give me a glass of Chardonnay, Ricky, and I'll be your sex slave forever," he said, laughing loudly.

"Oh, shut up, Darrell!" Nina cried. "Leave the poor boy alone. You're embarrassing him."

"*Moi*?" Darrell replied. "Would I do a thing like that? Just because I'd like to lick his face and suck his toes for a week is no reason for him to be embarrassed."

Mortified, the young bartender crept down to the opposite end of the bar and started polishing the wine glasses.

"Oh, Darrell, you're impossible!" Nina said, giggling. "You're a very bad boy. I don't know why I put up with you."

"Because you need me, darling."

"You're outrageous."

"And you love it! I always make you laugh."

"That's true," Nina admitted. "But sometimes you go too far."

"Too far?" Darrell snapped, in a tiff. "At least I'm not boring, like every other person in your perfect, lonely world. If I had any sense, I'd make you pay for my company. You can afford it, and I'm worth it."

"I always pick up the tab," Nina teased.

"You owe it to me, dearest. Don't I always listen to your pitiful little complaints and problems? If my problems were the size of yours I could fit them in a bud vase instead of a bunker." Darrell lowered his voice to a loud whisper. "And don't I always sit and talk to you until you're feeling better? Or until you're too drunk to feel anything at all? I can't even count how many times I almost lost my job because of you. The bookstore gives me an hour—not an entire afternoon—off for lunch.

"Which reminds me . . ." he went on. "I've got to get back to work in thirty-five minutes."

Nina didn't say anything. After a few seconds of silence, I took a sip of my club soda and snuck a quick glance in her and Darrell's direction. Still wearing her shades, Nina sat guzzling her drink while Darrell toyed with the stem of his wine glass. His large fingers looked like sausages.

"Everything's turned to shit," Nina finally mumbled. "I wish I was dead."

Darrell groaned. "What's happened *now*?"

"It's what *hasn't* happened that bothers me."

"What do you mean?"

"Oh, I don't know. It's nothing, really."

"Yeah? Nothing? Since when has nothing made you wish you were dead? C'mon, Nina. What gives? It's not like you to keep your troubles to yourself. You usually spray them all over the walls like graffiti."

"Oh, it's just the same old thing, Darrell. I'm ashamed to keep talking about it."

"Ashamed? I don't believe it. Darling, in all the years I've known you I've never even seen you blush. So what's the matter, honeyface? Niles acting up again?"

"No. He's not *acting* at all," Nina said, heaving a loud sigh. "That's the problem. He just sits in the white leather chair in the library, all day and all night, with his legs stretched out on the ottoman and his eyes closed. He even eats his meals there. The only time he took a shower and got dressed was for a magazine interview yesterday. And as soon as the interview was over, he went right back to his chair. That's where he was when I left to meet you. Vegetating in that goddamn chair."

"Well, look on the bright side, dearheart. At least you know where he is."

"Oh, shut up! Do you have to make a friggin' joke out of everything?"

"Of course I do! It's the only way I get through the day. If I didn't see life as one great big joke, I'd go take a nap on the subway tracks."

"Which line? The IRT or the BMT? I want to get a good seat."

Darrell's brawny laughter filled the room and rattled the liquor bottles. "That's better, darling! You're sounding like your old self again. The bitch you were born to be. So relax your beautiful bod and tell Daddy Darrell all about it. Why is Niles living in a chair? I was under the impression he preferred his office couch."

Nina giggled. "That was before his favorite patient and latest couchmate died," she said. "Remember? I told you about her. The super rich one who lived on a big estate in our neighborhood. The one Niles was obsessed with."

"She died?" Darrell gasped. He actually sounded shocked and upset. "What happened? Did Niles finally fuck up? Did she die on the operating table?"

"Christ, no! You've been watching too many goddamn soap operas."

"Well, I just thought—"

"Actually, she was murdered."

"What?" Darrell shrieked so loud I jumped and cracked my knee against the underside of the bar. "You don't mean it!" he cried. "When? How? Who did it?"

"Take it easy, baby," Nina said. "You look like you're going to have a coronary. It happened about a week ago. You must have seen it on TV or read about it in the papers. Her name was Jane Masterson. She was shot to death and her body was found in the trunk of a car at the Hempstead Library."

"Oh, yeah! I *did* read about that. Jane Camille Masterson. I remember her middle name because of the Greta Garbo movie. So *she* was your hubby's grand passion," he said in wonder. "They showed a picture of her in the newspaper. She was beautiful."

"Thanks to Niles," Nina said with an audible sneer.

"Whose car did they find the body in?"

"They didn't say. But the car owner wasn't the one who killed her."

"How do you know?"

"Because they would have arrested that person by now, Dumbo. For a girl, you're not so clever. Ever think of taking thinking lessons?" Nina teased.

But Darrell wasn't in the mood for jokes anymore. His voice had become hushed and serious. "So they still don't know who did it," he rasped. "But they must have some leads by now. Do they have any suspects?"

"How the hell should *I* know? The police don't keep me informed."

"Who would do such a horrible thing? Why would anybody want to kill a beautiful young girl like that?"

"Christ, Darrell! Will you please get that *I'm-so-shocked-and-sad* look off your face? You look like a moron! I don't buy your big concern act. And this conversation's getting really dull, too, so let's just drop the subject. I'm sorry I brought the whole thing up."

"Well, ex*cuuuse* me!" Darrell said. "Aren't we touchy! What's the matter *now*, darling?"

"Nothing. Let's get out of here. Come into Barneys with me. There's a blouse I'm thinking of buying, but I want your opinion first."

"I live to please you, dearheart," he said with a sniff. "And while we're in there, you can buy something for *moi*. Any little thousand-dollar trinket will do."

I turned my head and watched them walk toward the exit. Nina haughtily led the way and Darrell hobbled along behind her like a Saint Bernard on a too-short tether. When they reached the door, they both turned around to face the bar area again. "Bye-bye, Ricky!" Darrell called out to the bartender.

Nina shot a glance in Rick's direction and then her eyes fell on my face. She gazed at me for a couple of seconds through the dark green lenses of her sunglasses. I felt a sudden flush of anxiety, but quickly realized she didn't recognize me at all. In fact she hardly seemed to notice I was there. Darrell was equally unaware of my presence. To people like Nina and Darrell, mousy-looking, less than stylish middle-aged women are virtually invisible.

I paid for my club soda, tipped the bartender, and left the restaurant. I thought of going back into Barneys to continue spying on Nina, but my heart just wasn't in it anymore. Instead, I headed for home.

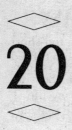

20

To drown out my jealous thoughts about Eddie and Claudine in Florida, I went straight for the vacuum cleaner. With clenched teeth and maniacal energy, I lugged the noisy beast around the house until every speck of plaster, dirt, and sawdust had been sucked into its bulging belly. Then I mopped the kitchen and bathroom floors and polished all the fixtures. I even did a load of laundry.

Nothing worked. My house was sparkling clean, but my mind was still filthy with fantasies. I watched Eddie and Claudine walking hand in hand down the beach at sunset; I saw them sharing a bottle of wine on the starlit balcony outside their hotel bedroom; I'm ashamed to admit I even looked on while they lay tanned and naked on their king-sized bed and rolled all over each other in breathtaking animal ecstasy. I was a mental wreck.

To keep from going totally insane, I gave Ellen a quick call to tell her I had finished the plastic surgeon interview and would be sending the article off to her in a few days. She was so grateful she promised to keep me in freelance work for the rest of my life. I didn't get too excited. For one thing, I didn't think she'd manage to hold on to her job that long—I figured another year, at the most. For another thing, I hoped I wouldn't be writing *Glamour*-ized bullshit for the rest of my life. I wanted to write a book someday. Something real and *meaningful*—like a murder mystery.

In the meantime, however, I had this plastic surgery article to do. And working on *that* seemed as good a way as any to get my mind off Eddie and Claudine. I turned on the Mac, opened up a new file and spent a half-hour or so transcribing the interview tape to type. Then I took out my handwritten notes, the Rebirth Center booklet, and my plastic surgery clip file and got down to business.

An hour and a half later I had put six solid pages of copy into the computer. Figuring that was enough for one day, I went into the kitchen to scrounge up some dinner. I put a piece of chicken and a baking potato in the oven and made a tomato and onion salad. Then I opened some wine, vowing to have just two glasses, *not* the whole bottle. While I was sipping the wine and waiting for my dinner to cook, I gave Philly a call.

"Lemme get this straight," Philly said after I told her about the events of the day. "You want me to quit my job and go to work for a crazy sex killer? That's one fine idea, girlfriend. Got anything else you want me to do? Like take a swim in a oil slick, maybe, or warm up my feet in the microwave?"

I laughed. "I know it sounds dangerous, but I really don't believe it would be. Think about it. If Ben *is* the murderer, they're bound to catch him sooner or later and put him away for life."

"Yeah, but what if it's later 'stead of sooner."

"Well, even if they don't catch him *at all*, it's not like he's a serial killer or anything, slaughtering people just for the fun of it. If Ben killed Jane, it was just so he would inherit all his father's money. He'd have no reason at all to want to kill you.

"Besides," I went on, "he has a new job in London and he's planning to move over there in two weeks. So, whether Ben's the murderer or not, he won't be living out at the Masterson estate anymore. He'll either be in Europe or in jail."

"Livin' in Europe don't mean nothin'," Philly insisted. "He's got more money than Oprah. He could fly home any ol' time he wants, and then he could bother my pretty brown ass all 'round the block and back. Too many black women been raped by white men already. I don't feel like havin' my name put in *that* book."

"First of all," I argued, "if he moves to London, he won't ever *want* to come home. He hates being around Bette and Daisy. Second of all, even if he *did* come back, and even if he *was* overcome with an uncontrollable desire to rape you, he'd never be able to succeed."

"Why not?"

"Because I'm sure that with all those years of lifting and moving old people in and out of beds and wheelchairs, you're much stronger than Ben." Having already thwarted two of Ben's attacks myself, I knew what I was talking about. "Not only that," I added, "you're much smarter than he is. He wouldn't stand a chance."

Philly giggled. It always made her feel good when I said she was smart. Probably because she still didn't really believe she was.

"Anyway," I went on, "have you forgotten how much

you hate working at the nursing home? Now's your chance to get out of that horrible, depressing place. And you wouldn't have to go into the dregs of Hempstead anymore. You could work in a lovely old mansion in a beautiful, safe neighborhood."

"Keep talkin' to me, girl," she said.

"You'd really like Bette and Daisy," I added. "They're great old gals. And you wouldn't have that much work to do, either. Bette sleeps a lot, so you'd have plenty of time to study for the licensed home health care aide test you're always talking about taking. I bet they'd even let me come over and give you reading lessons there, at the house—out on the patio or in the sunny breakfast room—during your working hours."

"Speakin' of workin' hours," Philly huffed, trying to hide her mounting interest, "what would they be? Five to ten years, with time off for good behavior?"

"Normal hours," I said. "Nine to five, Monday through Friday. Bette has somebody else to work the nights and weekends. And rush hour wouldn't be a problem because you'd always be driving in the opposite direction from most of the traffic. And, get this! You can have all your meals there, if you want to, free of charge. Breakfast and lunch—even dinner, if you feel like hanging around after work to eat with the family. Linda, the head maid, told me to be sure and tell you this. She said you could even live there, if you wanted to, in your own private room, but I told her you had your own life and you'd be going home to Woodrow."

"Hmmmm," Philly murmured, trying to sound doubtful instead of excited. "There's gotta be a big fat catch here somewhere. Like, what they gonna pay me? 'Bout fifty cents a hour?"

"Bette said that Dora, the woman who has the job now, is making $400 a week, plus coverage on the household medical plan. But I don't know what your salary would be. You'd have to meet with Ben and work that out with him."

"There's that ugly name, again," Philly moaned. "The bug in the bowl of soup."

"Who's being a scaredy-cat now? Are you going to let one little bug keep you from landing this dream job? This could be your first-class, one-way ticket out of nursing home hell. Take my word for it, Philly," I said with true conviction. "Ben won't be any threat to you at all." I gave her his phone number and urged her to call him right away.

"Oh, all right!" she finally agreed. "Lord, forgive me for bein' a damn fool! If I get raped and killed I hope you'll be able to live with your bad self! And just so's you'll never forget me, Annie, I'm gonna add a little somethin' extra to my will," she said, snickering. "I'm gonna put it down in *writin'* that Woodrow's got to have me cremated and scatter my ashes in your car trunk."

I ate my dinner, watched TV for a while, and got ready to go to bed early. After a long hot shower, I put on my freshly washed stuck-out-tongue T-shirt and crawled between my clean white sheets. I hoped I would fall asleep fast and forget all about what Eddie and Claudine might be doing in *their* bed.

No such luck. I couldn't sleep and I couldn't stop imagining things. I was so tightly wound up that when the doorbell first sounded, my body sprang up in the air and almost splattered against the ceiling. With the taste of fear in my mouth, I vaulted out of bed and grabbed hold of one of my pillows. Hugging it in front of me for protection—Perfect! A shield of feathers!—I crept into the dark living room.

The doorbell rang again. Careful not to make a sound, I slunk over to the window nearest the door and gently pried a peephole in the venetians. Peering out, I came eyeball to bloodshot eyeball with somebody else peering *in*!

I squealed and jumped back from the window. My chest tightened up and I couldn't breathe. My first impulse was to dash back into the bedroom and hide under the covers, but I quickly stifled that notion. I didn't want to act like a wuss anymore. I wanted to act like Wonder Woman. Still clutching the pillow to my breast, I lurched forward, grabbed the cord to the venetians and yanked it all the way down. The blinds flew up and locked at the top, leaving the picture window, and the man standing in the light on the front porch, fully exposed.

I looked at the man's face and my heart leaped into my throat. It was Eddie. And he didn't look the least bit tan. He looked tired, disheveled, and so startled he had crouched to go for his gun. I was so happy to see him I lunged for the front door, flipped the two locks, and pulled the door wide open. This set off the alarm, of course, and the shocking, earsplitting shrieks of the siren sent us both into total meltdown.

The following events were like scenes from a Three Stooges movie. Eddie pulled his gun, held it out in front of him with both hands, and started pouncing around on the porch, pointing the damn thing in all directions. Berserk and barefoot, I tripped out onto the porch, anxiously dropped my pillow to the floor, and then scrambled back into the living room to punch wildly at the alarm system number pad.

Detecting my sudden movements behind his back,

Eddie wheeled around, saw my big white pillow billowing unexpectedly in the breeze, and quickly aimed his gun at it, as any trained professional would do. At that precise moment, one of my cats ran yowling out of the house and—tail frizzed up like a Christmas tree—streaked right between his legs. Eddie stumbled out of position, cracked his knee against one of my wrought iron porch chairs, and pitched forward. The chair tumbled over and Eddie went with it, falling toward the floor with both hands still gripping the gun—which accidentally went off, discharging a bullet smack in the middle of my pillow.

The blast was deafening. A big cloud of feathers burst into the air and then slowly disseminated, each little feather wafting toward its own private landing place. Eddie struggled to his feet and I moved closer to the door. We both stared at the frothy spectacle with bulging eyes and open mouths while the alarm continued to howl. I heard the phone ringing in the background, but I didn't answer it. Finally, after what seemed like a weekend but was just a few seconds, some small measure of sense returned to my head and I remembered my secret alarm code. I punched the numbers into the system and we were blessed with sudden silence.

I poked my head out the door and looked at Eddie. He looked back at me in total amazement. Then, as the stunning realization of what had just happened came over us, we smiled at each other, chuckled a little bit, and shook our heads in awe. Faces contorted with mirth and wonder, we watched the last few floating feathers settle to the ground. Eddie walked toward the door and stared down at the charred, fluffy mess that had once been my pillow.

"Is it dead?" I asked him.

He laughed and put his gun away. Then he walked into the house and took me in his arms.

Before I knew what I was doing, I had slipped my hands inside the front of Eddie's open jacket and snaked my arms below his shoulder holster and around his back. I stood up on my bare tiptoes, wound my arms more snugly beneath his jacket and—trembling with lust and joy—pressed my chest against his warm shirt-front. I gave no thought to my actions. I sought out the heat and smell and safety of Eddie's body like a mind-less, mewling kitten.

Eddie moaned and pulled me closer. His heart beat like a conga drum against my breasts. He pushed one hand up under my hair and clasped the nape of my neck. Then he gathered up a fistful of hair and gently pulled my head back, away from his shoulder. He looked down into my eyes, released a soft growl from the back of his throat and kissed me full on the mouth.

I think I actually lost consciousness for a moment. It was as if my soul had been sucked out and swallowed up. When the blood returned to my brain, Eddie wasn't kissing me anymore. He was stroking my face with his fingers and smiling.

"I've wanted to do that since the night we met," he said.

"Mmmph skooch," I replied. It's hard to speak intel-ligibly when your lips are in shock.

"Are you okay?" he asked me.

"No!" I cried, moving away from him and staggering toward the couch. My legs were so wobbly I had to sit down.

"What's the matter?" he asked, sitting down next to me.

I didn't know what to say. Every emotion known to woman was raging through my body like a hurricane. "I thought you were in Florida," I mumbled.

"I just got back tonight. I came here straight from the airport."

"How's the weather down there?" *Get a grip, Annie. Would Wonder Woman sit there like a wimp and ask about the weather?*

"Huh? Oh, I don't know. Sunny, I guess."

"How's the family?" I asked. *Translation: How's your beautiful, big-breasted wife?*

"They're okay," he said, sighing. "The kids aren't too happy about being yanked out of school again, but I think they'll be all right. They'll be coming back up here next month to spend the summer with me."

"What?"

"They'll spend the summer with me and go back to live with Claudine in the fall, when school starts."

"I don't understand," I said. "Aren't you moving to Ft. Lauderdale?"

"God, no! What gave you that idea?"

"Well, when they said you were in Florida, I just naturally thought—"

"You've got it all wrong," Eddie broke in. "*I'm* not moving to Florida, *Claudine* is. She ran into her old high school boyfriend when she was in Indiana—he was there visiting his sick father—and they fell for each other all over again. He's a rich dentist in Ft. Lauderdale and he's got a big house on the beach. He's been divorced twice.

"Anyway," he went on, "John—that's his name, John—asked Claudine to move down there with the kids and live with him, and she decided to do it. She just didn't tell *me* about it. She came back home, but *not to* try to patch things up between us, like I thought. All that talk about me getting a new job and us moving to Florida was a smoke screen. She was just keeping me at arm's length while she made arrangements for *herself* and the *kids* to move. And while she was at it, she made arrangements to get a legal separation from me."

"How considerate of her."

"Yeah," he said, rubbing his face. "Claudine doesn't mess around. When she makes her mind up about something, it's a done deal."

"Did you go down there to try to change her mind?"

"No. I'm ready for the marriage to end. We've both been pretty miserable for a long time. I'm just worried about the kids. I went down there to see where they would be living and to make sure they're all right."

"And are they?"

"Yeah, I think so. John's a nice enough guy and he seems to like them a lot. He took Kevin to a baseball game and bought Annette a music box."

"You'll miss them terribly," I said.

"Every minute," he agreed.

"Will you miss Claudine?" I asked.

"Like a toothache," he said.

Light from the porch streamed into the dark living room through the picture window behind the couch, giving us both a golden glow. Eddie put his right arm around me and softly rubbed the side of my neck. "I wasn't kidding about what I said before, Annie," he murmured. "I know it sounds crazy—I mean, we've known each other for such a short while—but I'm really nuts about you. I think about you all the time."

His words shot a current of electricity down my spine and actually made my mouth water. I wanted him so much I could taste it.

Placing one hand on each of my shoulders, Eddie pulled my upper body toward his and began grazing his fingers up and down my arms. Then, out of the blue, he asked, "What's that shirt you're wearing?"

"It's my Rolling Stones T-shirt," I said, laughing. "It's what I sleep in. Don't you like it?"

"Not much," he admitted.

"Then I'll take it off," I said. Breathless with my own boldness, I tucked my fingers under the hem of the T-shirt, pulled it up over my bare breasts, and tossed it on the coffee table. Brave actions, I thought, for a middle-aged broad who hadn't been naked in front of a man for over five years. *Wonder Woman rides again!*

Eddie gasped and pulled me closer to him on the couch. Hungrily moving his hands over my bare back and shoulders, he covered my face and mouth with hot kisses. Then he slid his hand up my side, under my arm, and enveloped my naked breast with his big warm fingers.

That was when I heard the police sirens. They came screaming around the distant corner and wailed all the way up the street, whining to a stop right in front of my house. With a sick feeling in the pit of my stomach, I realized why they were there.

"It's the cops!" I cried, forgetting that I was talking to one. "They're answering the alarm. They think somebody broke into the house!"

"Shit!" Eddie muttered, gulping for air. He removed his sweet hands from my body and began straightening his jacket.

I felt suddenly cold. "I'd better get some clothes on!" I jumped to my feet and dashed into my bedroom. Pulling on a sweatshirt and a pair of jeans, I rejoined Eddie in the living room as quickly as I could.

Everything that happened next kind of merged into a blur. I hopped around the living room turning on lights while Eddie met the local policemen at the door. He showed them his badge and identification and told them there was nothing for them to worry about, there had been a false alarm. But the police weren't convinced. And—homicide detective or no—they wouldn't take Eddie at his word. The fact that my front lawn was carpeted in feathers, and the smell of gunpowder was wafting in the air, and there was a hole as big as Boston blasted in my porch floor, probably had something to do with their suspicion.

They wanted to see my driver's license, or something with my address on it to prove that I actually lived there, and they wanted to check out the rest of the "domicile." Four of Rockville Centre's finest tromped into my little house and plodded from room to room, looking for signs of illegal entry and God knows what other criminal activities. Then they went out the back door and combed the back yard looking for clues to who knows what else. All they found were a few more goose feathers—it was a breezy night.

Eventually, after Eddie talked to the police for a while—telling them he was at my house in the line of duty, working on the Masterson rape and murder case—they started to back off. They asked about the hole in the porch floor, and Eddie told them his gun had gone off accidentally. Then, after asking a few questions about the murder and how the investigation was going, they finally left—without ever learning the cause of the plumage proliferation.

And Eddie was left standing in the middle of my living room with his passion gone and his tail between his legs. He was overcome with shame. It didn't matter that it was just a pillow, he said, or that shooting it had been a freak accident. He *never* should have let such a thing happen. The skeptical looks on the faces of the other policemen had made him realize how dangerous and irresponsible his conduct had been. He had acted wildly, and he deserved to have his badge and his gun taken away. The fact that he was emotionally and physically exhausted from his Florida trip and family problems was no excuse. He had been trying to protect me, but he might have *killed* me, and he never would have been able to live with that. How could he ever, *ever* have fired his gun so recklessly? He wasn't worth the paper his numerous citations were printed on.

Hoping to make him feel better, I said everything I could think of to minimize the incident. But Eddie wasn't having any. He just wanted to go home, he said. He needed to be alone. He'd call me tomorrow. He rested his lips on my cheek for a second and stepped out on the porch.

Then, suddenly squatting down near the edge of the porch, he started fishing around in the border ferns with his hands. He had to find the spent cartridge and its casing, he explained, to turn in to headquarters, along with a full report on when and how and why he fired his gun. Finally locating the battered shell and its covering, he stood up and sheepishly put them in his pocket. Then, trying not to look at the hole in the floor or the feathers on the lawn, he left.

As soon as Eddie's car disappeared around the corner, I realized I'd forgotten to give him the coin purse full of Ben's hair. I was surprised at my memory lapse, but with everything happening the way it did, the murder had been the last thing on my mind.

I called my lunatic cat back inside, locked up the

house, and went into the bedroom. Then I took off my clothes and put my T-shirt back on. As I crawled back into bed, I couldn't help thinking how much easier it was going to be to fall asleep *now* than it had been earlier—now that I could dream about Eddie making love to *me* instead of Claudine. I turned out the light, put my head down on the spare pillow, and lay there grinning from ear to ear in the dark.

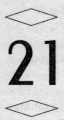

21

I spent a large portion of the next morning plucking feathers off the grass and out of the bushes, ignoring the ones that had blown into the neighbors' yards or gotten snagged in the treetops. Then I cleaned up the shattered slate and cement around the pothole in the porch floor. After discarding a trash bag full of gravel and feathers in the garbage bin at the side of the house, I went back indoors and forced myself to work on the plastic surgery article.

It wasn't easy. I didn't feel like writing. I felt like lounging in bed naked, eating chocolates, and reading love comics. I wanted to close my eyes and let my mind drift in rich, sweet daydreams about Eddie. Writing about breast implants and butt tucks was a poor substitute. I managed to get through it, though, printing out two copies of the finished article before lunchtime. After wolfing down a bowl of vegetable soup and a handful of crackers, I called the Stanwyck residence.

"*Whom* shall I say is calling," the maid replied when I asked for Dr. Stanwyck.

"Annie March from *Glamour* magazine."

"Ooooh!" she cooed, suddenly sounding like a starstruck girl of twelve. "Hold the line, please. I'll see if he's in."

It was a full five minutes before anyone picked up the phone again. "This is Nina Stanwyck," said the bored voice at the other end. "Can I help you?"

"Hi, Nina. This is Annie March from *Glamour*. I've finished the article on your husband and I was wondering if I could drop by today and bring the manuscript for him to read over. I promised him full copy approval."

"Couldn't you just fax it?"

"I don't have a fax machine," I lied. "And he has to sign a release. I'm up against a *very* tight deadline and I need to get his approval today."

"Oh, all right," she said, with a sigh of annoyance. "Come to Niles's office at two o'clock."

"Thanks. I'll be there." I made a face at the phone and hung up.

It was a very warm day so I changed out of my sweats into a short denim skirt, black V-neck T-shirt, and a pair of sandals. I put a Billie Holiday album on the stereo, went into the bathroom and sang "Love For Sale" to the mirror while I put on some makeup. I was dabbing on a coat of Honey Ginger lipstick—and thinking about Eddie kissing me—when he called.

"Hi," he said in his deep yummy voice. My insides started purring.

"Hi," I answered with enough warmth to melt the mouthpiece.

"I'm sorry about last night," he said. "I really messed up."

"No you didn't!" I insisted. "You were my hero! You were wonderful. A bit like Don Quixote," I said, giggling, "but wonderful just the same."

Eddie laughed. "Windmills are more respectable opponents than pillows. I'd rather talk about some of the *other* things that happened last night," he went on, with a sinfully suggestive smile in his voice, "but I can't right now. This call is for business, not pleasure. There's been a break in the Masterson case, and Lieutenant O'Donnell wants to see you this afternoon. Would that be possible?"

"What happened?" I cried. "What did you find out? Do you know who the killer is?"

"Not yet, but we're getting close. And that's all I can tell you right now. Can you come into headquarters later?"

"I could get there by four or four-thirty. Would that be all right?"

"That'll be fine. O'Donnell's due in at three. He usually doesn't come in on Saturday, but he's making an exception for you."

"I can't stand it! You've *got* to tell me what's going on! Am I going to be arrested or something?"

"No," he said, chuckling. "That much I *can* tell you. You're not even a suspect anymore."

"Really? Then you must know who the murderer is! Why can't you tell me? Just give me the initials," I begged.

"We really *don't* know who the killer is yet, Annie. I wouldn't lie to you. But now I've got to go. Got another call coming through. I'll see you at four. You'll find out everything then. And I'll take you to dinner afterward, okay?"

"Okay." I yielded with heightened, but mixed emotions. I was furious at Eddie for not telling me what was going on, but I still couldn't wait to lay eyes—and, hopefully, hands—on him again.

I decided to take Ben's hair sample into headquarters with me instead of waiting to give it to Eddie when we were alone. If I really wasn't a suspect anymore, I could stop worrying about how the cops might perceive my actions, or my easy access to the evidence. I wondered if I should cancel my appointment with Niles Stanwyck; if I should put my personal investigation on hold until I found out everything the cops had learned. But, since I needed to get the article approved and delivered to Ellen anyway, I figured I might as well follow through on my earlier plans.

I went back into the bathroom to finish putting on my lipstick. I gave my hair a good brushing and fluffed it with my fingers. By the time Billie started keening the lovesick lyrics to "Body and Soul," I was ready to hit the trail.

Even nature bows to the wealthy. As I drove into the heart of Sands Point, the lush shade tree shelter caused an eight to ten degree drop in the temperature—a significant improvement over the record 92 degrees registered by the mercury in the *real* world that morning. The cooler air was moist instead of muggy, and—thanks to Sands Point's acres and acres of flowering shrubs and towering evergreens—noticeably less polluted. I filled my lungs with the wonderful stuff.

The maid met me at the entrance to the downstairs office and—mouth stretched into an impossibly wide smile—showed me inside. "Please have a seat," she said, batting her lashes so ferociously I thought they might fly off her face. "I'm afraid Dr. Stanwyck won't be able to see you today. He's very busy. He wants you to wait here in the office while I take the article upstairs for him to read. Is that okay?"

"Sure," I said, handing her the manila envelope which contained the manuscript and release and smiling to hide my disappointment. I had hoped to talk to Niles long enough to sneak in a few more questions about Jane. I had even stuck my tape recorder in my purse on the off chance he might have something interesting—or incriminating—to say.

"I'll take the article up to him now," the maid said, opening a door at the back of the office. From my seat in the side chair near the desk, I could see that the door led to a staircase, which obviously led up to the main floor of the house. "Can I get you something to drink?" she asked before heading upstairs. "Some lemonade or some iced tea?"

"No, thank you. I'll be fine."

As soon as she left, I got up and started snooping around the office. If I couldn't get more information about Jane by talking to Niles, at least I could poke around for some other kinds of clues. First I checked out the floor-to-ceiling bookcase behind the desk. Nothing but some leather-bound medical tomes, some hardcover plastic surgery books, a TV set and VCR, a few paperbacks about nutrition and fitness and lots of slick new books about beauty, body image, makeup, and skin care. No family photos or personal items.

I was about to start looking through the desk drawers when I heard someone clomping down the stairs from the main level of the house. I bolted around the desk and sat back down in my chair before the office door opened and Nina walked in. She was wearing a yellow and black satin kimono and black satin platform mules—hence the Frankenstein footfalls on the stairs.

As she walked across the thick gray office carpeting, her shoes slapped loudly against the soles of her feet.

"You'll have to wait your turn," she said, coming to a stop in front of my chair and sneering down at me from her lofty platforms. "Niles is having a manicure right now and he can't read your article until his nails are dry. He'll try to get to it right after that, unless the hairstylist arrives, in which case you'll have to wait even longer. Niles takes his glasses off when he's getting a haircut, so he can't read until it's finished. I'm sorry for the delay, but it can't be helped. There's an important charity ball at our country club tonight and we both have a lot of preparations to make."

"I understand," I said in a voice so sweet it made me squirm. "And don't worry about me. I don't mind waiting at all. It'll give me a good chance to check out the competition," I said, gesturing toward the stack of women's fashion magazines sitting on the coffee table by the couch.

Nina sniffed and looked at her watch. "It's time for my massage." She shot a look of annoyance in my direction and turned her back on me. "I'll send the maid down with the article when he's read it," she said, tossing her words over her shoulder like little wads of cellophane trash.

"Thanks," I said. It took some effort, but I managed to keep the word *bitch* in my head and off my tongue.

Nina flip-flopped her way to the door and clomped back up the stairs. I sat still as a statue till the coast was clear. Then I darted back behind the desk, settled down in Niles's black leather chair and slowly pulled open the top right desk drawer. I was breathing normally and my heart was keeping a regular beat. My palms were dry instead of sweaty. Somehow, sometime during the past week I had grown accustomed to playing this detective game.

The object I found sitting on a stack of stationery in

the very back of the desk drawer, however, almost made me wet my pants. It was a gun. A sleek and streamlined stretch limo of a gun. A huge and hideous killer shark of a gun. It was black, about seven or eight inches long, and it looked like it would weigh at least three pounds—but I couldn't say for sure, since I didn't pick it up. Pick it up? God, I wouldn't even *touch* the damn thing! Not because I was afraid of smudging existing fingerprints, or leaving behind some new ones of my own, but because I was afraid of shooting myself in the foot.

I sat staring into the drawer for several long, airless seconds—wondering if this was the gun that killed Jane; wondering if the gun that killed Sam was as big and ugly as this one; wondering if I should force myself to grab the hateful thing, stash it in my purse and take it with me to police headquarters for ballistic evaluation. I didn't know what to do.

Finally, after gaping at the gun for another minute or two, I eased the drawer closed and returned to my chair on the other side of the desk. For some reason I felt that the best course of action was *in*action. I needed time to think. I snatched a magazine off the coffee table and started flipping through its pages so I would look occupied when the maid came back downstairs.

My eyes were on the pictures, but my mind was on the murder. And my crowded thoughts were racing around my brain like wild horses around a dog track. Maybe I had been all wrong about everything from the beginning. Maybe Ben hadn't raped *or* killed his half sister. Maybe Niles had shot Jane when he found out she was having an affair with another man. Another *married* man. A man whose name and number Jane *wouldn't* have written in her Filofax. A man so concerned with secrecy he couldn't let himself attend his own lover's funeral.

It was an all-too-possible scenario, I realized. And now it even struck me as the *most likely* scenario. Jane could have broken up with Niles, telling him she was in love with someone else and then driving off to meet her new paramour. Crazy with jealousy, Niles could have decided to kill Jane, feeling he had a creator's *right* to destroy his own creation. Maybe he waited for nightfall, grabbed the gun out of his desk drawer, and drove over to the Masterson estate in a rage.

Finding Jane just returned from her lovers' tryst, down on her knees in her pink T-shirt and gray sweatpants working in the greenhouse, Niles could have simply walked over to her and—with one little squeeze of one manicured finger—blown her away forever. And if that was what had happened, then Jane might not have been raped at all. It might have just *looked* like rape since she had had sexual intercourse right before she was murdered.

It all kind of fell into place and made semilogical sense, except for a couple of things: why were Jane's clothes cut to pieces? And how did her body wind up in my car trunk?

I was staring at a layout of Calvin Klein swimsuits, searching for an answer to those burning questions, when the maid returned with my manuscript. "Dr. Stanwyck read your article, and he signed the release. The magazine can print it just like it is."

"Good." I stood up and took the envelope from her, folding it in half and stuffing it into the side pocket of my shoulder bag. "Thanks for your help."

"You're *very* welcome," she simpered, eyelashes aflutter. "My name's Dotty, and if there's ever anything *else* I can do for you, just let me know."

"Well, it's nice to finally know your name, Dotty," I

said, smiling broadly and extending my hand for her to shake. "Sorry to be a nuisance on such a busy day. What's all the activity about anyway?" I asked, pretending total ignorance.

"Oh, they're going to a big dinner dance at their club tonight, and everything's got to be just perfect. The doctor's pretty much finished with his personal appointments for the day, but Mrs. Stanwyck still has a seamstress, a hairstylist, and a makeup artist coming. She already had her pedicure, manicure, leg-waxing, and massage."

"That's a lot of preening for one night out," I said. "Sounds like Mrs. Stanwyck has read too many *Glamour* magazines."

Dotty laughed as if that was the funniest thing she'd ever heard in her life, but she didn't really mean it. She was buttering me up big time. What did she think I was going to do for her? Get her a free lifetime subscription? Give her a job modeling lingerie? Put her somewhat pretty face on the cover? Whatever fantasies were floating in that dotty little head of hers, I decided to play along. It could pay to have a friend in the enemy camp.

"Well, I guess I'll be going now," I said, pulling my purse over my shoulder and heading for the office exit. "It was nice to meet you, and I hope to see you again someday."

"Oh, me too!" she cried, opening the door for me. She smoothed out the skirt of her pink and gray uniform, hit me with another beaming smile and started flapping her lashes again. For one awful second I thought she was going to curtsy.

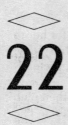

22

Late afternoon sun poured through the window of Lieutenant O'Donnell's office, forming a large golden patch on the ugly green carpet. O'Donnell's forehead was beaded with sweat and his silver hair clung damply to his large cranium. In spite of the heat, his shirt collar was securely buttoned and his tie was snugly noosed around his neck.

"Don't they give you any air-conditioning in here?" I asked.

"It's too early in the season," he said. "They don't turn it on till the middle of June. Come hell or high water."

"Or a freak heat wave," Eddie added, standing near the door and blotting his own forehead with one of his light blue shirtsleeves. Even in his wilted clothes and steamy discomfort, he looked sublime.

I sat anxiously in the brown leather side chair—the same chair I had squirmed in the week before, when I first learned I was a suspect in the case and overheard the two officers discussing the rape and murder of Jane Camille Masterson. I wasn't being grilled this time, at least, but the air was just as stifling and I still felt like I was in the hot seat. Literally. The backs of my legs kept sticking to the leather and every time I moved there was an embarrassing sucking sound.

"So what's the story?" I asked, unable to wait for O'Donnell to bring up the subject himself. "Have you caught the murderer? Am I off the hook now?"

"We don't know who the murderer is," the Lieutenant said simply, "but we *have* caught the rapist. And, yes, you *are* off the hook now."

"Who? What? How?" I sputtered in my usual calm and dignified manner.

"The rapist was arrested at the Masterson estate yesterday afternoon," O'Donnell answered, "and we've obtained a full confession."

Poor Ben, I thought. Conked by a lamp after breakfast, then cuffed by the cops after lunch. An altogether unpleasant day. The first in a long, punishing series of unpleasant days, I hoped.

"I don't understand," I said. "He confessed to raping her, but not to killing her? That doesn't make sense. He had a real *motive* for killing her."

"What motive would that be?" Eddie asked me.

"The money, of course. Full and exclusive title to all the Masterson millions."

Both men stared at me blankly for a few seconds. Then they looked at each other and smiled. "She's got the right string," O'Donnell said to Eddie, "but the wrong yoyo."

"What do you mean?" I asked.

"Ben Masterson didn't rape his sister," Lieutenant O'Donnell said. "Juan Lopez did."

"Who?"

"Juan Lopez," Eddie repeated. "The gardener at the Masterson estate."

"Oh!" I blurted, head reeling. "Juan! I *knew* he was hiding something, but I thought he was just protecting Ben—keeping secrets for his boss so he could keep his job. He looked *terrified* the day I was snooping around the greenhouse. Is that where Jane was raped? In the greenhouse?"

"You got it," Eddie said, with a nod in my direction. "Down on the floor, fifth aisle over from the door."

"But that's where she was shot!" I cried. "So Juan *must* have been the one who killed her, too. He raped her and then shot her so she wouldn't ever be able to tell anybody."

"That's not the way it happened," Eddie said softly.

"How do you know?" I asked.

"Because Juan Lopez didn't have a gun, or any access to a gun," Lieutenant O'Donnell answered. "And because Jane Masterson was already dead when he raped her."

I felt like someone had kicked me in the stomach. Raped *after* she was murdered? The thought was intolerable—even more intolerable than the thought of a normal rape—if any rape could *ever* be called *normal*. With a loud sob of anguish, I squeezed my eyes shut and covered my face with both hands. Then I mashed my fingertips deep into my eye sockets, trying to stop the sickening visions from taking shape in my brain.

It didn't work. The horror movie started rolling, flashing one grisly image after another: Jane's blood-soaked clothes being cut away from her lifeless form with a pair of hedge clippers; her poor flesh being mauled by callused and dirty hands; her helpless body being mounted by a deranged animal in a red plaid workshirt. And through it all, Jane's eyes—those astonishingly empty eyes!—staring glassily at the greenhouse ceiling, seeing nothing.

Eddie walked over to the side of my chair and put his hand on my shoulder. "Are you okay?" he asked.

"Yes," I said, but I wasn't. I felt like throwing up.

"It's not a pretty picture," O'Donnell said in a burnt-out tone of voice that suggested he'd seen worse. Much worse.

"At least she didn't *know* she was being raped," Eddie said, trying to console me. And that thought *did* make me feel a little better. That and the feel of Eddie's firm hand on my shoulder.

"How do you know she was already dead?" I asked.

"The Medical Examiner has his ways," O'Donnell said.

"We've known it all along," Eddie added.

"Was Juan there when the murder took place? Did he see or hear anything?"

"He was in the adjoining room," Eddie said, "but his door was closed. He heard the gun go off, but he was too chicken to go out and see what was happening. He just cowered near the door for a while, listening at the crack, waiting to see if anything else was going to take place. He thought he heard somebody run out and slam the greenhouse door, but he can't say for sure. By the time he finally got up the nerve to go into the green-house, there was nobody there. Nobody but Jane, and she was definitely dead."

"So he just waltzed right over to the tool rack, grabbed the goddamn pruning shears, cut off all her clothes, and raped her?"

"Something like that," O'Donnell muttered.

"It's too horrible!" I cried. "How *could* he?"

"Seems he's been obsessed with Jane since he first started working at the Masterson estate seven months ago," Lieutenant O'Donnell said. "Thought she had a great body. Whenever she was working out in the gardens or in the greenhouse, he watched her every move. He says she always wore a loose, low-necked T-shirt and no bra at all. He couldn't take his eyes off her. He would hide and peer through the bushes at her, waiting for her to bend over and give him a good look. And he could never get enough.

"So," the Lieutenant continued, "when he saw her lying there on the greenhouse floor—his for the taking, with nobody around to see—something just snapped. He couldn't help himself, he said. He *had* to have her."

"He's full of remorse now, though," Eddie said. "Ever since we brought him in he's been crying like a baby. He's ashamed for his wife and six kids, he says. We had to put him on suicide watch."

"You should've loaned him your razor instead," I said.

A few minutes later Detective Lou Hobbs stuck his basset hound face into the office and gave me a rubbery smile. "Hi, Toots," he said.

"Hi!" I said, happy to see his trusty mug.

"Can I talk to you a minute, boss?" he said to Eddie. "We got a new lead on the Jefferson boy's death."

Eddie frowned and blotted his forehead again. "Be back in a few minutes," he said, turning to follow Hobbs out.

I watched Eddie walk away and then turned to O'Donnell. "So, I'm not a suspect anymore, right? What else did you find out?" I asked. "What put me in the clear?"

"We found out how the body wound up in your car trunk."

"*How?*" I cried.

"Juan Lopez put it there."

"Juan? But why? He doesn't even know me. Why would he want to implicate me? Did Ben put him up to it?"

"Ben didn't put him up to it, and Juan didn't want to implicate you. In fact, the whole thing had nothing to *do* with *you*."

"Then, why—"

"If you'll just relax and stop asking so many questions, I'll *tell* you why," O'Donnell blustered, his face turning red. The heat was getting to him.

"Sorry," I said meekly. "You talk, I'll listen."

"Good." He raked his fingers through his hair and adjusted his shirt collar. "It's pretty simple, really. After Lopez raped the body, he got scared. He thought somebody would find out what he did, and he thought he'd be blamed for the murder, too. So, in a desperate effort to cover *all* the tracks, he shoved Jane's body and clothes into a heavy-duty lawn and leaf bag, wheelbarrowed the bag out to the parking area and loaded it into the back of his truck. Then he hosed down the area of the greenhouse where Jane was killed and repaired the damaged floor runner with a spare section from the storage shed.

"Lopez wasn't worried about anybody in the house looking out the window and seeing what he was up to," O'Donnell went on. "He knew it would look like he was just doing normal chores. He was anxious to get rid of the body, though. So he cleaned up the greenhouse as fast as he could and left the estate in a big hurry.

"Then he *really* panicked. He didn't know what to do with the body. He was afraid to stop and dump it anywhere by the road. There was a lot of traffic that night and the chances were too great that he'd be seen. So, like the total asshole he is—pardon my language— he drove all the way home with the body still in the back of his truck. Then he started driving around the streets near his apartment building looking for a place to hide it.

"It had started raining, so there weren't any people out walking around. And the Hempstead Library parking lot was deserted. He pulled into an empty parking space, jumped out of the truck and started looking for an unlocked car trunk.

"As luck would have it," the Lieutenant said, giving me an apologetic smile, "his truck was parked right next to your car and your trunk was the first one he tried to open. Not only was it unlocked, but it was big and it was *empty*. Lopez pulled out of the parking spot, backed up to your car's rear end and then just *rolled* the body out the back of his truck into your open trunk. It was a piece of cake."

"Ugh!" I groaned.

"Right," he said.

"And you have a full confession?"

"Taped, typed, and signed."

"Including the part about my car trunk?"

"Including the part about your car trunk, which was covered with Lopez's fingerprints. And while we're on the subject," he added, "I hope you'll accept my apology for any inconvenience we may have caused you during the course of this investigation."

I gave him a weak smile. "You were just doing your job, right?"

"Right," he grunted.

"So, can I get my car back now?"

"Sorry," he said. "The case isn't closed yet. We'll have to keep your car until the murderer is arrested and tried."

"And how soon will that be?" I asked. "You must have a lead suspect by now."

"I'm not at liberty to discuss it," he said, sticking to the rule book like a fanatic Boy Scout. "And, while we're on that subject, let me say I hope—the whole *department* hopes—that you'll butt out now and leave the rest of this investigation up to us. We know you've been playing detective, Mrs. March, looking for evidence to prove your own innocence. And we can understand your need to get involved—in spite of all the extra trouble you've caused us. But now that you're no longer under suspicion, I must insist that you stop sticking your nose into this case. It would be very dangerous and stupid for you to get more entangled than you already are. I assure you the NCPD will catch the killer soon, and we'll do it much more easily *without* your help than with it."

In light of his nasty attitude—and since the rapist had already been nailed—I decided not to give O'Donnell the hair sample in my purse. I didn't tell him about the gun I saw in Niles Stanwyck's office, either.

"There's still one thing I don't understand, Lieutenant," I said. "The library is just a few feet away from the Hempstead Police Station. How could Juan have risked unloading the body there? Wasn't he scared of being seen by the police? He could have been arrested on the spot!"

"We asked him about that. He said he didn't know the police station was there."

"But that's crazy!" I insisted. "How could he *not* know? I guess it's possible he didn't see all the squad cars—it was dark and they're parked in a different lot. But how could he have missed the huge stationhouse sign? It's all lit up and it says Police as big as day."

"I can answer that one," O'Donnell said. "The son of a bitch can't read."

23

In B.K. Sweeney's the air was cold and my martini was icy. But the fact that Eddie was sitting across the table from me, sprawling lazily in his chair and looking as gorgeous and sexy as any man ever had a right to look, kept my body heat set on sizzling. In an effort to act cool and casual, I plucked an olive out of my martini and sucked the pimento from its center. Then I leaned forward.

"So what do you make of it?" I probed, stuffing the rest of the olive into my mouth and chewing it to a salty pulp. "Who's wearing the black hat now? Who do you think the murderer is?"

Eddie gave me a slow, sweet smile and sat up closer to the table. "You know I can't talk about that, Annie."

"Why not?" I whined. "I'm not a suspect anymore! You don't have to worry about clueing me in on any secret police stuff. Can't you just talk about the case with me the way you would with any interested friend?"

"Your interest goes way beyond friendly," he said,

with a stern parental tone in his voice. He looked so cute I wanted to lean over the table and kiss every freckle on his face.

"My detective days are over," I declared. "Now that I'm not trying to dodge a bum murder rap, I can return to my dull civilian life."

"I wish I could believe that."

"You *can* believe it!" I insisted, widening my eyes into giant orbs of innocence. I was trying to resemble Little Orphan Annie, but I probably looked more like Daisy Duck. "That doesn't mean I'm not still dying to know who did it, however. And under the circumstances, I think my curiosity is completely understandable."

Eddie didn't say anything. He just stared at me for a few seconds, trying to see inside my head, sizing me up in the same way he might scrutinize an unreliable witness. Then he glanced around the crowded restaurant, lifted his hand in the air, and summoned a waiter to our table. Giving the menu a quick once-over, he ordered grilled swordfish and a salad. I ordered spaghetti.

"So what do you think?" I continued as soon as the waiter left our table. "Did Ben do it? At one point I was positive he was the killer, but now I'm not so sure. He certainly had the clearest motive, but Niles Stanwyck had the means."

"What are you talking about?" Eddie said, cocking his head to one side and staring at me again.

"I'm talking about the gun in the doc's desk drawer," I blurted. It was nasty of me to just spit it out like that. Whether the cops had already found the gun or not, I knew it would upset Eddie to learn that *I* had discovered its existence. But I had my reasons for being so blunt. I wanted Eddie to think I wasn't hiding anything anymore, and I wanted to get a rise out of him—get him talking about the case.

"Okay," he said, annoyed. "I'll bite. How do you know about the gun?"

"I saw it today, while I was alone in Niles's office, waiting for him to read the article I wrote about him for *Glamour* magazine. I was looking around for a pencil and I just happened to—"

"Yeah, right!" Eddie broke in. "And the dog ate your homework. What else did you *just happen* to find in the drawer? A signed confession, maybe?"

"No," I said, smiling. "But the fact that Niles has a gun *is* sort of suspicious don't you think? I mean, it bears looking into, wouldn't you say?"

"Jesus, Annie! When are you going to wake up?" Eddie whacked the top of the table in exasperation. "The NCPD is *not* as slow and stupid as you like to think. Niles Stanwyck turned his gun over to us last Saturday, the same day we questioned him about the murder. It was checked out by our ballistics experts and—although it's the same *kind* of gun that killed Jane Masterson—every single test proved it was *not* the murder weapon."

Combing his fingers through his curly hair, Eddie leaned back in his chair again. "We had no reason to keep the gun for evidence," he went on, "so we returned it to Dr. Stanwyck a couple of days later. And he, I assume, returned it to his desk drawer—just in time for you to *just happen* to find it."

"Oh," I said, at a loss for words.

"And what's this about you doing a magazine article on Stanwyck?" Eddie asked. "That's a clever little investigative ploy. How did you manage that one?"

"A friend of mine is an editor for *Glamour*," I explained, trying to look like Little Orphan Annie again,